Robert Dale Owen

Moral Physiology

A brief and plain treatise on the population question

Robert Dale Owen

Moral Physiology
A brief and plain treatise on the population question

ISBN/EAN: 9783742833594

Manufactured in Europe, USA, Canada, Australia, Japa

Cover: Foto ©Lupo / pixelio.de

Manufactured and distributed by brebook publishing software (www.brebook.com)

Robert Dale Owen

Moral Physiology

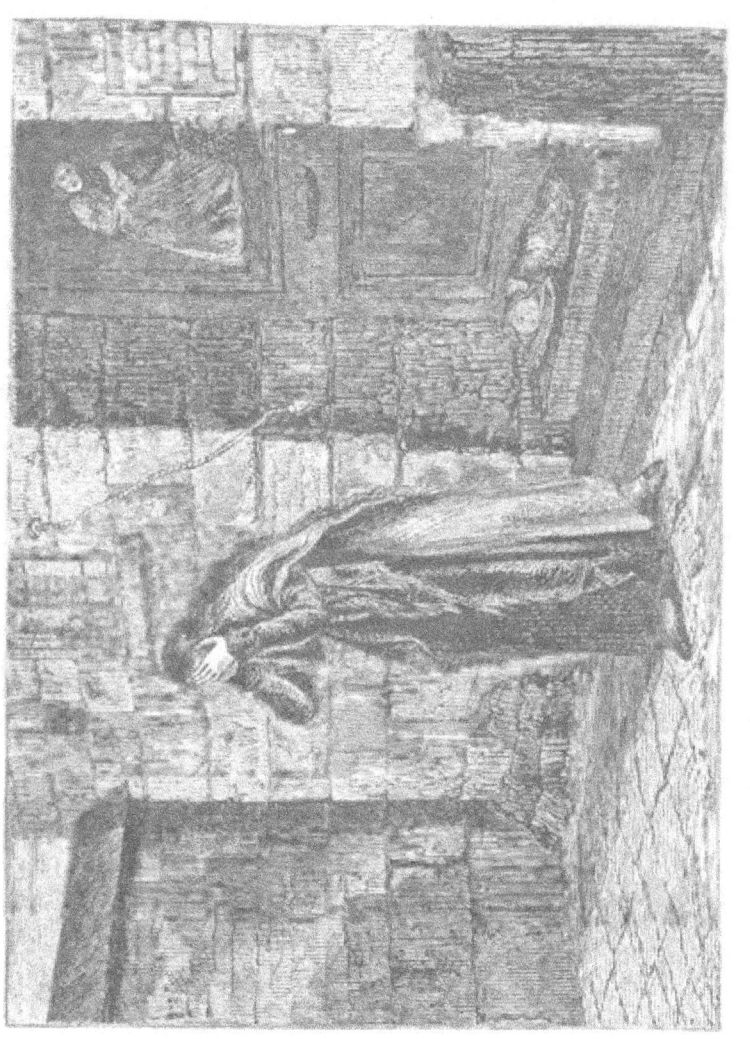

Alas! that it should ever have been born!

MORAL PHYSIOLOGY;

OR,

A BRIEF AND PLAIN TREATISE

ON THE

POPULATION QUESTION.

BY ROBERT DALE OWEN.

The principle of utility is the foundation of the present work.
Bentham on Morals and Legislation.

TENTH EDITION, **WITH NOTES BY THE** PUBLISHER,
bodying all Modern Discoveries—illustrated by Anatomical and Physiological Engravings.

BOSTON:
PUBLISHED BY J. P. MENDUM,
AT THE OFFICE OF THE "BOSTON INVESTIGATOR."
1875.

*. The frontispiece which accompanies this treatise, represents a poor mother abandoning her infant, at the gate of the Hôtel des Enfans trouvés, (Foundling Hospital) at Paris. The original painting, from which this is a faithful copy, is by Vigneron, a French artist of celebrity; it was purchased at the price of one thousand dollars for the Galerie Royale, and is now in the possession of the French king.

The Hôtel des Enfans trouvés, than which a more humane institution was never founded, exhibits, in its every arrangement, order, economy, and, above all, a beautiful tenderness of the feelings of those poor creatures who are thus compelled to avail themselves, for their offspring, of the asylum it affords. No obtrusive observation is made, no unfeeling question asked: the infant charge is received in silence, and either trained and supported until maturity, or, if circumstances, at any subsequent period, enable the parents to claim their offspring, it is restored to their care.

There is surely no sect, of creed so frozen, or ritual so rigid, that it can systematize away the common feelings of humanity, or dry up, in the breasts of some gentler spirits, the milk of human kindness. The benevolent founder and indefatigable supporter of this noble institution was a Jesuit! Be the good deeds of St. Vincent de Paul remembered, long after the intrigues and cruelties of his fellow sectaries are forgotten!

The case selected is one of mild, of modified,—I had almost said, of *favoured* misfortune: an extreme case were too revolting for representation. But even under these comparatively happy circumstances, when benevolence extends her Samaritan care to the destitute and the forsaken, who that regards for a moment the abandoned helplessness of the deserted child, and the mute distress of the departing mother, but will join in the exclamation "Alas! that it should ever have been born!"

PREFACE.

It may be proper to state, in few words, the immediate circumstances which induced me, at the present time, to write and publish this treatise.

Some weeks since, a gentleman coming from England brought with him two pretty specimens of English typography. One represented a triumphal arch with a statue of the late king, and was made up of 17,000 different pieces of common printing type; the other, an altar piece, having the Lord's Prayer, Creed, and Commandments, printed within it, and composed of about 13,000 separate pieces. The gentleman was requested by a Brighton printer who executed them, to present these, as specimens of English typography, to some of his brethren craftsmen in America. He presented them to me; I admired the ingenuity displayed in the performance; but thought they ought to have been presented rather to some printers' society than to an individual. I therefore addressed them to our Typographical Society in New-York, accompanied by a note simply requesting the society's acceptance of them, as specimens of the art in England.

I thought no more of the matter, until I received, the other day, my specimens back again, with a long and not a little angry letter, signed by three of the members, accusing Robert Dale Owen of principles subversive of every virtue under heaven, and calculated to lead to the infraction of every commandment in the decalogue: and, more especially, accusing him of having given his sanction to a work, as they expressed it, "holding out inducements and facilities for the prostitution of their daughters, sisters, and wives."

I subsequently learned, from one of the society, circumstances which somewhat extenuate (albeit nothing can excuse) their childish incivility. A gentleman who busied himself last year in making out a notable reply to the "Society for the Protection of Industry," got up, at a late Typographical meeting, and read to the Society several detached extracts from a pamphlet written by Richard Carlile, entitled "Every Woman's Book," which extracts he pronounced to be excessively indecent; and asked the Society whether they would receive any thing at the hands of a man who publicly approved a book of a tendency so dreadfully immoral; which, he averred, I had done. The society were (or affected to be) much shocked, and thereupon chose a committee to return to me the heretical specimens, which committee penned the letter to which I have alluded.

Probably some members of the society really did believe the work to be of pernicious tendency. Had some garbled extracts only from it been read to me, I might possibly have utterly misconceived its tone and tendency, and its author's motives. But he must be blind indeed, who can read the pamphlet through, and then (whether he approve it or not) can attribute other than good intentions to the individual who was bold enough to put it forth.

As to the book itself, I was requested, two years since, when residing in Indiana, to publish it, and declined doing so. My chief reasons were, that I doubted its physiological correctness; that I did not consider its style and tone in good taste; but chiefly (as I expressed it in the New Harmony Gazette) because I feared it would be circulated in this country only "to fall into the hands of the thoughtless, and to gratify the curiosity of the licentious, instead of falling, as it ought, into the hands of the philanthropist, of the physiologist, and of every father and mother of a family." The circumstances I have just detailed may afford proof, that my fears regarding the hands into which it might fall, were well founded.

My principles thus officiously and publicly attacked, I have felt it a duty to the cause of reform to step forward and vindicate them; and this the rather, because, unless I give my own sentiments, I shall be understood as unqualifiedly endorsing Richard Carlile's. Now, no one more admires than I do the courage and strength of mind which induced that bold advocate of heresy to broach this important subject; and to him be the praise accorded, that he was *the first* to venture it. But the manner of his book I do not admire. There is in it that which was repulsive (I will not say revolting) to my feelings, on the first perusal; and though I afterwards began to doubt whether that first impression was not attributable, in a great measure, to my prejudices, yet I cannot doubt that a similar, and even a more unfavourable impression, will be made on the minds of others, and thus the interests of truth be jeopardized. Then again, I think the physiological portion of his pamphlet somewhat incorrect as to the facts, and therefore calculated to mislead, where an error might be of fatal consequence.

It may seem vanity in me to imagine, that this treatise is free from similar objections; yet I have taken great pains to render it so.

R. D. O.

P. S. (*to the fourth edition.*) Communications from intelligent individuals, on whose physiological knowledge I place reliance, have enabled and induced me somewhat to modify the text, and alter the arrangement, of the sixth chapter.

MORAL PHYSIOLOGY.

I sit down to write a little treatise, which will subject me to abuse from the self-righteous, to misrepresentation from the hypocritical, and to reproach even from the honestly prejudiced. Some may refuse to read it; and many more will misconceive its tendency. I would have delayed its publication, had the choice been permitted me, until the popular mind was better prepared to receive it. but the enemies of reform have already foisted the subject, under an odious form, on the public; and I have no choice left. If, therefore, I prematurely touch the honest prejudices of any, let them bear in mind, that the occasion is not of my seeking.

The subject I intend to discuss is strictly a physiological subject, although connected, like many other physiological subjects, with political economy, morals, and social science. In discussing it, I must speak as plainly as physicians and physiologists do. What I mean, I must say. Pseudo-civilized man, that anomalous creature who has been not inaptly defined "an animal ashamed of his own body," may take it ill that I speak simply: I cannot help that.

A foreign princess, travelling towards Madrid to become queen of Spain, passed through a little town of the peninsula, famous for its manufactory of gloves and stockings. The magistrates of the place, eager to evince their loyalty towards their new queen, presented her, on her arrival, with a sample of those commodities for which alone their town was remarkable. The major domo, who conducted the princess, received the gloves very graciously; but, when the stockings were presented, he flung them away with great indignation, and severely reprimanded the magistrates for this egregious piece of indecency. "Know," said he, "that a queen of Spain has no legs."*

I never could sympathize with this major domo delicacy; and if you can, my reader, you had better throw this pamphlet aside at once.

If you have travelled and observed much, you will already have learnt the distinction between real and artificial propriety. If you have been in Constantinople, you probably know, that when the grand seignor's wives are ill, the physician is only allowed to see the wrist, which is thrust through an opening in the side of the room, because it is improper even for a physician to look upon another man's wife; and it is thought better to sacrifice health than propriety.†

If you have sojourned among the inhabitants of Turcomania, you know that they consider a woman's virtue sacrificed for ever, if, before marriage, she be seen to stop on the public road to speak to her lover:‡ and if you have read Buckingham's travels, you may remember a very romantic story, in which a young Turcoman lady, having thus forfeited her reputation, is left for dead on the road by her brothers, who were determined their sister should not survive her dishonour.

Perhaps you may have travelled in Asia. If so, you cannot be ignorant how grossly indecorous to Asiatic ears

---

* See "Memoires de la Cour d'Espagne," by Madame d'Aunoy.
† See Tournefort's Travels in Turkey.
‡ See Buckingham's Travels in Asia.

it is, to enquire **of a** husband after his wife's health; and probably you **may know,** that **men have** lost their lives to atone for **such an impropriety.** You know, too, of course, **that in Eastern nations it** is indecent for a woman **to uncover her face ; but perhaps you may not know, unless your** travels have extended **to Abyssinia, that there the** indecency consists **in uncovering the feet.***

In Central Africa, you may have seen **women bathing** in public, without the slightest sense of impropriety; **but** you were doubtless told, that men could not be **permitted a similar liberty ; seeing that modesty requires they** should **perform their ablutions in private.**

If my reader has **seen all or any of these countries** and customs, I doubt not that he or she will read my little book understandingly, and interpret it **in the purity which springs** from enlarged and enlightened views ; or, indeed, from common sense. If not—if you who now peruse **these lines have been educated at** home, and have never passed the boundary **line of** your own nation— perhaps **of your own** village—if **you have not** learnt that there **are other** proprieties besides those of your **country ; and** that, after all, genuine modesty has its legitimate seat in the heart rather than in the outward form or sanctioned custom—then, I fear me, you **may** chance to cast these pages from you, as the major domo did **the proffered stockings, unconscious that the indelicacy lies, not in my simple** words, or the Spanish magistrates' **honest offering, but in the pruriently** sensitive **imagination that discovers** impropriety in either. Yet, even though unexperienced, if you **be** still young and pure-minded, **you may** read this pamphlet through, and I shall fear from **your lips,** or in **your** hearts, no odious misconstruction.

* See Bruce's Travels in Abyssinia.

Young men and women! you who, if ignorant, are uncorrupted also; you in whose minds honest and simple words call up none but honest and simple ideas; you who think no evil; you who are still believers in human virtue and human happiness; you who, like our fabled first parents in their paradise, are yet unlearned alike in the hypocritical conventionalities and the odious vices of pseudo-civilization; you, with whom love is stronger than fear, and the law within the breast more powerful than that in the statute book; you whose feelings are still unblunted, and whose sympathies still warm and generous; you who belong to the better portion of your species, and who have formed your opinion of mankind from guileless spirits like your own—young men and women! it is to your pure feelings I would fain speak: it is by your unsophisticated hearts I would fain have my treatise and my motives judged.

Libertines and debauchees! this book is not for you. You have nothing to do with the subject of which it treats. Bringing to its discussion, as you do, a distrust or contempt of the human race—accustomed as you are to confound liberty with licence, and pleasure with debauchery, it is not for your palled feelings and brutalized senses to distinguish moral truth in its purity and simplicity. I never discuss this subject with such as you. It has been remarked, that nothing is so suspicious in a woman, as vehement pretensions to especial chastity: it is no less true, that the most obtrusive and sensitive stickler for the etiquette of orthodox morality is the heartless rake. The little intercourse I have had with men of your stamp, warns me to avoid the serious discussion of any species of moral heresy with you. You approach the subject in a tone and spirit revolting alike to good taste and good feeling. You seem to presuppose—from your own experience, perhaps—that the hearts of all men, and more especially of all women, are deceitful above all things and desperately wicked; that violence and vice are inherent in human nature, and that nothing but laws and ceremonies prevent **the world** from becoming a vast slaughter-house or a universal brothel. You judge your own sex and the other by the specimens you have met with in wretched haunts of mercenary profligacy; and, with such a standard in your minds, I marvel **not that you remain** incorrigible unbelievers **in any virtue,** but that which is forced, on the prudish hot-bed of ceremonious orthodoxy. **I** wonder not, that you will not trust the natural soil, watered from the free skies and warmed by the life-bringing sun. How should you? you have never seen it produce but weeds and **poisons.** Libertines and **debauchees! cast** my book aside! You will find in it nothing to gratify a licentious curiosity; **and, if you** read it, you will probably only give me credit for motives and impulses like your own.

And you, prudes and hypocrites! you **who** strain at gnat and swallow a camel; you whom Jesus likened to **whited** sepulchres, which without indeed are beautiful, but within are full of all uncleanness; you who affect to blush if the ancle is incidentally mentioned in conversation, or displayed in crossing **a style,** but will read in**decencies enough, without scruple, in** your closets; **you** who, **at dinner, ask to be helped to the bosom of a duck,** lest, by mention of the word breast, you call up improper associations; **you who have nothing but a** head and feet and fingers; **you who look demure by** daylight, and make appointments **only in the dark—you,** prudes and hypocrites! I do not address. Even if honest in **your** prudery, your ideas of right and wrong are too artificial and confused to profit by the present discussion; if dishonest, I desire to have no communication with you.

Reader! if you belong to the class of prudes or of libertines, I pray you, follow my argument no farther. Stop here, and believe that my heresies will not suit you. As a prude, you would find them too honest; as a libertine, too temperate. In the former case, you might call me a very shocking person; in the latter, a quiz or a bore.

But if you be honest, upright, pure-minded; if you be unconscious of unworthy motive or selfish passion; if truth be your ambition, and the welfare of our race your object—then approach with me a subject the most important to man's well-being; and approach it, as I do, in a spirit of dispassionate, disinterested, free enquiry. Approach it, resolving to prove all things, and hold fast that which is good. The discussion is one to which it is every man's and every woman's *duty*, (and ought to be every one's *business*,) to attend. The welfare of the present generation, and—yet far more—of the next, requires it. Common sense sanctions it. And the national motto of my former country, "Honi soit qui mal y pense,"* may explain the spirit in which it is undertaken, and in which it ought to be received.

Reader! it ought to concern you nothing who or what I am, who now address you. Truth is truth, if it fall from Satan's lips; and error ought to be rejected, though preached by an angel from heaven. Even as an anony-

* One of the English kings, Edward III., in the year 1344, picked up from the floor of a ball-room, an embroidered garter belonging to a lady of rank. In returning it to her, he checked the rising smile of his courtiers with the words, "Honi soit qui mal y pense!" or, paraphrased in English, "Shame on him who invidiously interprets it!" The sentiment was so greatly approved, that it has become the motto of the English national arms. It is one which might be not inaptly nor unfrequently applied in rebuking the mawkish, skin-deep, and intolerant morality of this hypocritical and profligate age.

mous work, therefore, this treatise ought to obtain a full and candid examination from you. But, that you may not imagine I am ashamed of honestly discussing a subject so useful and important, I have given you my name on the title page.

Neither is it any concern of yours what my character is, or has been. No man of sense or modesty unnecessarily obtrudes personalities that regard himself on the public. And, most assuredly, it is neither to gratify your curiosity or my vanity, if I now do violence to my feelings, and speak a few words touching myself. I do so, to disarm, if I can, prejudice of her sting; and thus to obtain the ears, even of the prejudiced; and also to acquaint my readers, that they are conversing on such a subject as this, with one, whom circumstance and education have happily preserved from habits of excess and associations of profligacy.

All those who have intimately known the life and private habits of the writer of this little treatise, will bear him witness, that what he now states is true, to the letter. He was indebted to his parents for habits of the strictest temperance—some would call it abstemiousness —in *all* things. He never, at any time, habitually used ardent spirits, wine, or strong drink of any kind: latterly, he has not even used animal food. He never chanced to enter a brothel in his life; nor to associate, even for an evening, with those poor, unhappy victims, whom the brutal, yet tolerated vices of man, and sometimes their own unsuspicious or ungoverned feelings, betray to misery and degradation. He never sought the company but of the intellectual and self-respecting of the other sex, and has no associations connected with the name of woman, but those of esteem and respectful affection. To this day, he is even girlishly sensitive to the coarse and ribald jests in which young men think it witty to indulge at the expense of a sex they cannot appreciate. The confidence with which women may have honoured him, he has never selfishly abused; and, at this moment, he has not a single wrong with which to reproach himself towards a sex, which he considers the equal of man in all essentials of character, and his superior in generous disinterestedness and moral worth.

I check my pen. I have said enough, perhaps, to awaken the confidence of those whose confidence I value; and enough, assuredly, to excite the ridicule, or the sneer, of him who walks through life wrapped up in the cloak of conformity, and laughs, among his private boon companions, at the scruples of every novice, who will not, like himself, regard debauchery and seduction (in secret) as manly and spirited amusements.

And now, reader! if I have succeeded in awakening your attention and enlisting in this enquiry your reason and your better feelings, approach with me a subject the most interesting and important to you, to me, to all our fellow-creatures. Reader! if you be a woman, forget that I am a man: if a man, listen to me as you would to a brother. Let us converse, not as men, nor as women, but as human beings, with common interests, instincts, wants, weaknesses. Let us converse, if it be possible, without prejudice and without passion. Reader! whatever be your sex, sect, rank, or party, to you I would now, ere I commence, address the poet's exhortation—here, far more strictly applicable, than in the investigation to which he applied it:—

> " Retire! the world shut out: thy thoughts call home.
> Imagination's airy wing repress.
> Lock up thy senses; let no passion stir:
> Wake all to reason; let her reign alone."

CHAPTER II.

STATEMENT OF THE SUBJECT.

Among the human instincts which contribute to man's preservation and well-being, the instinct of reproduction holds a distinguished rank. It peoples the earth; it perpetuates the species. Controlled by reason and chastened by good feeling, it gives to social intercourse much of its charm and zest. Directed by selfishness, or governed by force, it is prolific of misery and degradation. Whether wisely or unwisely directed, its influence is that of a master principle, that colours, brightly or darkly, much of the destiny of man.

It is sometimes spoken of as a low and selfish propensity; and the Shakers call it a " carnal and sensual passion."* I see nothing in the instinct itself that merits such epithets. Like other instincts, it may assume a selfish, mercenary, or brutal character. But, in itself, it appears to me the most social and least selfish of all our instincts. It fits us to give, even while receiving, pleasure; and, among cultivated beings, the former power is ever more highly valued than the latter. Not one of our instincts, perhaps, affords larger scope for the exercise of disinterestedness, or fitter play for the best moral

---

* See " A brief exposition of the principles of the United Society called Shakers," published by Calvin Green and Seth Y. Wells, 1830.

feelings of our race. Not one gives birth to relations more gentle, more humanizing and endearing; not one lies more immediately at the root of the kindliest charities and most generous impulses that honour and bless human nature. Its very power, indeed, gives fatal force to its aberrations; even as the waters of the calmest river, when dammed up or forced from their bed, flood and ruin the country: but the gentle flow and fertilizing influence of the stream are the fit emblems of the instinct, when suffered, undisturbed by force or passion, to follow its own quiet channel.

That such an instinct should be thought and spoken of as a low, selfish propensity, and, as such, that the discussion of its nature and consequences should be almost interdicted in what is called decent society, is to me a proof of the profligacy of the age, and the impurity of the pseudo-civilized mind. I imagine that if all men and women were gluttons and drunkards, they would, in like manner, be ashamed to speak of diet or of temperance.

Were I an optimist, and, as such, had I accustomed myself to judge and to admire the arrangements of nature, I should be inclined to put forward, as one of the most admirable, the arrangement according to which the temperate fulfilling of the dictates of this, as well as of almost all other instincts, confers pleasure. The desire of offspring would probably induce us to perpetuate the species, though no gratification were connected with the act. In the language of the optimist, then, "pleasure is gratuitously superadded." But, instead of pausing to admire arrangements and intentions, the great whole of which human reason seems little fitted to appreciate or comprehend, I content myself with remarking, that this very circumstance (in itself surely a fortunate one, inasmuch as it adds another to the sources of human happiness) has often been the cause of misery; and, from a blessing, has been perverted into a curse. Enjoyment has led to excess, and **sometimes to tyranny and barbarous injustice.**

Were the reproductive instinct disconnected from pleasure of any kind, it would neither afford enjoyment nor admit of abuse. As it is, the instinct is susceptible either; just as wisdom or ignorance governs human laws, habits, and customs. It behooves us, therefore, to **be especially careful in its** regulation; else what is a great good may become for us a great evil.

This instinct, then, may be regarded in a two-fold light; *first*, as giving the power of reproduction: *secondly*, as affording pleasure.

And here, before I proceed, let me recall to the reader's mind, that it is the province of rational beings to bear UTILITY strictly in view. Reason recognizes as little the romantic and **unearthly reveries of Stoicism, as she** does the doctrines of health-destroying and mind-debasing debauchery. She reprobates equally a contemning and an abusing of pleasure. She bids us avoid asceti**cism on** the one hand, and excess on the other. In all our enquiries, then, let reason guide us, and let UTILITY be our polar star.

I have often had long arguments with my friends, the **Shakers,* touching the** two-fold light **in which the reproductive instinct may be regarded.** They commonly **stand** out stoutly against the propriety of considering it **except simply as** a means of perpetuating the species;

---

* I call them my friends, because, however little **I am disposed to accede** to all their principles, I have met, from among **their body, a greater** proportion of individuals who have taken with them **my friendship and sympathy, than perhaps from among any other sect or class of men** and, apart from that, they deny that it may be regarded as a legitimate source of enjoyment. In this I totally dissent from them. It is a much more noble, because less purely selfish, instinct, than hunger or thirst. It is an instinct that entwines itself around the warmest feelings and best affections of the heart; and, though it differ from hunger and thirst in this, that it may remain ungratified without causing death, **I have** yet to learn, that because it is *possible*, it is therefore also *desirable*, to mortify and repress it. I admit, to the Shakers, that in the world, profligate and hypocritical as we see it, this instinct is the source of infinite misery; perhaps even, on the whole, **of** a *balance* of unhappiness: and I always freely admit to them, that if I had to choose between the **life of** the profligate man of the world and that of the ascetic Shaker, I should not hesitate a moment to prefer the latter. But, for admitting that the most social and kindly of human instincts is sensual and degrading in itself, I cannot. I think its influence moral, humanizing, polishing, beneficent; and that the social education of no man or woman is fully completed without it. Its mortification (though far less injurious than its excess) is yet very mischievous. If it do not give birth to peevishness, or melancholy, or incipient disease, or unnatural practices, at least it almost always freezes and stiffens the character, by checking the flow of its kindliest emotions; and not unfrequently gives to it a solitary, antisocial, selfish stamp.

I deny the position of the Shaker, then, that the instinct is justifiable (if, indeed, it be at all) only as necessary to the reproduction of the species. **It is justifiable** in my view, just in as far as it makes man **a happier and a** better **being**. **It is** justifiable, both as a source of temperate enjoyment, and as a means by which the sexes can mutually polish and improve each other.

If a Shaker has read my little book thus far, and cannot reconcile his mind to this idea, he may as well shut it at once. I found all my arguments on the position, that the pleasure derived from this instinct, independent of and totally distinct from, its ultimate object, the reproduction of our race, is good, proper, **worth securing and enjoying**. I maintain, that its **temperate enjoyment is** a blessing, both in itself **and in** its influence on **human character**.

Upon **this distinction of** the instinct into its two-fold **character**, hinges the chief point in the present discussion. It sometimes happens, nay, it happens every day and hour, that mankind obey its **impulses, not from any calculation of consequences, but** simply from animal impulse. Thus many **children that are brought into the** world owe their existence, **not to deliberate conviction in** their **parents that their birth was really** desirable, but **simply to an unreasoning instinct, which men,** in the **mass, have not learnt either to resist or control.**

It is a serious question—and **surely an** exceedingly **proper and** important one—whether man can obtain, **and** whether he is benefitted by obtaining, control over this instinct. Is **IT DESIRABLE, THAT IT SHOULD NEVER BE GRATIFIED WITHOUT AN INCREASE TO POPULATION? OR, IS IT DESIRABLE, THAT, IN GRATIFYING IT, MAN SHALL BE ABLE TO SAY WHETHER OFFSPRING SHALL BE THE RESULT OR NOT?**

To answer the questions satisfactorily, **it** would be necessary to substantiate, **that such** control may be obtained without the slightest **injury to** the physical health, or **violence to the** moral feelings; and also, that it should be obtained without any real sacrifice of enjoyment ; or, if that cannot be, with as little as possible.

Thus have I plainly stated the subject. It resolves itself, as my readers may observe, into two distinct heads: first, the *desirability* of such control; and, secondly, its *possibility*.

In discussing its desirability, I enter a wide field, a field often traversed by political economists, by moralists, and by philosophers, though generally, it will be confessed, to little purpose. This may be, in a great measure, **attributed** rather **to** their fear than their ignorance. The world would not permit them to say what they knew. I intend that my readers shall know all that I know on the subject; for I have long since **ceased to ask** the world's leave to say what I think, **and what I believe to** be useful to the public.

I propose to begin by considering the question in the abstract, and then to examine it in its political and social bearings.

CHAPTER III.

THE QUESTION EXAMINED IN THE ABSTRACT.

Is it in itself desirable, that man should obtain **control** over the instinct of reproduction, so as to determine when its gratification shall produce offspring, and when it shall not?

But that common sense is so scarce an article, and that the various superstitions of the nursery pervade the opinions and cramp the enquiries, even of after life—but for this, the very statement of the question might suffice to obtain for it the assent of every rational being. Nothing so elevates man above the brute creation, as the power he obtains over his instincts. The lower animal follows them blindly, unreflectingly. The serpent gorges himself; the bull fights, even to death, with his rival of the pasture; the dog makes **deadly war for a bone.** They know nothing of progressive **improvement.** The elephant or the beaver of the nineteenth century, are just as wise, and no **wiser, than** the elephant or the **beaver** of two thousand years ago. Man alone has the power to improve, cultivate, elevate his nature, from generation to generation. He alone can control his instincts by reflection of consequences, and regulate his passions by the precepts of wisdom.

It is strange, that even at this period of the **world, we** should have to remind each other, that *all* knowledge of facts is useful; or, at the least, cannot be injurious. The knowledge of some facts may be unimportant; the knowledge of none is mischievous. A human being is a puppet—a slave, if his ignorance is to be the safeguard of his virtue. Nor shall we know where to stop, if we follow up this principle. Shall we give our sons lessons in mechanics? but they may thereby learn to pick locks. Shall we teach them to read? but they may thus obtain access to falsehood and folly. Shall we instruct them in writing? but they may become forgers.

Such, in effect, was the reasoning of men in the dark ages. When Walter Scott puts in the mouth of Lord Douglas, on the discovery of Marmion's treachery, the following exclamation, it is strictly in accordance with the spirit and prevailing opinions of the times:

> " A letter forged! Saint Jude to speed!
> Did ever knight so foul a deed!
> At first in heart it liked me ill,
> When the king praised his clerkly skill.
> Thanks to Saint Bothan, son of mine,
> Save Gawain, ne'er could pen a line:
> So swore I, and so swear I still,
> Let my boy bishop fret his fill."

But the days are gone by when ignorance may be the safeguard of virtue. The *only* rock-foundation for virtue is knowledge. There is *no* fact, in physics or in morals, that ought to be concealed from the enquiring mind. Let that parent who thinks to secure his sons' honesty or his daughters' innocence by keeping back from them facts—let that parent know, that he is building up their morality on a sandy foundation. The rains and the floods of the world's influence shall beat upon that virtue, and great shall be the fall thereof.

If man, then, can obtain control over this most important of instincts, it is, *in principle,* right that he should know it. If men, after obtaining such knowledge, think fit not to use it ; if they deem it nobler and more virtuous, to follow each animal impulse, like the beasts of the field and the fowls of the air, without a thought of its consequences, or an enquiry into its nature —then let them do so. The knowledge that they have the power to act more like rational beings, will not injure, if it fail to benefit them. They are at perfect liberty to set it aside, to neglect it, to forget it, if they can. Only let them show common sense enough to permit that others, who are more slow to incur sacred responsibilities, and more willing to give reason the control of instinct, should obtain the requisite knowledge, and follow out their prudent resolutions.

If this little book were in the hands of every adult in the United States, not one need profit by it, unless he sees fit. Nor will any man admit that he can possibly be injured by it. Oh no. *His* virtue can bear any quantity of light. But then, his neighbour's, or his son's, or his daughter's!

This would lead me to discuss the *social bearings* of the question. But, as conceiving it more in order, I shall first speak of it in connexion with political economy.

CHAPTER IV.

THE QUESTION IN ITS CONNEXION WITH POLITICAL ECONOMY.

The population question, as it is called, has of late years occupied much attention, especially in Great Britain. It was first prominently brought forward and discussed, through two large volumes, by Malthus, an English clergyman. Godwin, Ricardo, Thompson, Place, Mill, and other celebrated cotemporary writers, have all discussed it, with more or less reserve, and at greater or less length.

Malthus' work has become the text book of a large politico-economist party in England. His doctrine is, that "*population, unrestrained, will advance beyond the means of subsistence.*" He asserts, that in most countries population at this moment presses against the means of subsistence; and that, in all countries, it has a tendency so to do. He recommends, as a preventive of the growing evil, celibacy till a late age, say thirty years; and he asserts, that unless this "moral restraint" is exerted, vice, poverty and misery, will and must become the checks to population. His book, in my opinion, has done infinite mischief. I have heard his disciples openly declare, that they considered the crimes and wretchedness of society to be *necessary*—to be the express ordainings of Providence, intended to prevent the earth from being over-peopled. I have heard it argued by men of rank, wealth and influence, that the distinctions of rich and poor, and even of morality and immorality, of luxury and want, will and must exist to the end of the world; that he who attempts to remove them fights against God and nature; and, if he partially succeed, will but afford the human race an opportunity to increase, until the earth shall no longer suffice to contain them, and they shall be compelled to prey on each other. It must be confessed, that this is a comfortable doctrine for **the rich idler: it is a healing** salve to **the luxurious conscience; an** opiate to drown **the** still **small voice of truth and humanity, which calls to every man to be up and do his part towards the alleviation of the human suffering that every where stares him in the face.**

It **is vain to argue with these** defenders of the **evils** that be, **that the day of overstocking is afar off.** They tell **you,** it must come at last; **and that the more you do to remove vice and misery—those** destroyers of **population—the sooner it** will come. **And** what reply can one make to the argument in the abstract? I believe it to be proved, that population, unrestrained,* will double itself **on** an average every twenty-five to fifty years. If so, it is evident to a demonstration, that, if population **be not** restrained, morally or immorally, the **earth** will *at last* **furnish no** foothold for the **human beings that will cover it.**

Take a medium calculation as to the natural rate of

---

* By *unrestrained*, Malthus and his disciples mean, not restricted or destroyed by any incidental check whatever, moral or immoral, prudential or violent. Thus, poverty, war, libertinism, famine, &c. are all powerful checks to population. In this sense, and not simply as applying to preventative moral restraint, have I employed the word throughout this chapter.

increase, and say, that population, unrestrained, will double itself every *thirty-three and a third* years. That it has done so, (without reckoning the increase from emigration,) in many parts of this continent, is certain.

Then, if we suppose the present numerous checks to population, viz. want, war, vice, and misery, removed by rational reform, and if we assume the present population of the world at one thousand millions, we shall find the rate of increase as follows:

At the end of 100 years, there will be 8,000 millions.
——————— 200 ——————— 64,000 ———
——————— 300 ——————— 512,000 ———
——————— 400 ——————— 4,096,000 ———
——————— 500 ——————— 32,768,000 ———

And so on, multiplying by 8 for every additional hundred years. So that, in 500 years, there would be more than *thirty thousand* times as many as at present: and in 1000 years, upwards of *a thousand million* times as many human beings as at this moment: consequently, *one single pair*, if suffered to increase without check, *would, in* 1000 *years, increase to more than double the present population* **of the** *globe.*

It appears evident, then, to a demonstration, that population **CANNOT be suffered to** increase unrestrained for more than a very few hundred years. **We are thus compelled** to admit to Malthus, that, *sooner or later,* some restraint or other to population *must* be employed; and compelled to admit to his aristocratic disciples, that if no other better restraint than vice and misery can be found, then *vice and misery must be;* they are the lot of man, from generation to generation.

Let me repeat it: it is no question—never can be a question—whether there shall be a restraint to population or not. There **MUST** be; unless indeed we find the means of **visiting other planets, so as to** people them. In the nature of things, there must be a check, of some kind, at some time. The *only* question is, what that check shall be—whether, as heretofore, the check of war, want, profligacy, misery; or a "moral restraint," sanctioned by reason and suggested by experience.

Let those, then, who cry out against this little treatise, be told, that though they may postpone the question, no human power can evade it. It must come up. Had the friends of reform been left to choose their own time, it might, perhaps with advantage, have been postponed. And it is an imaginable case, that prejudice might delay it until a general famine or a universal civil war became the frightful checks. But will any man of common sense argue the propriety of suffering such a crisis to approach?

Malthus saw this. He saw that some check must exist; and, whatever some of his disciples might permit themselves to say, he did not choose to be considered the apologist of vice and misery. His theory, indeed, supplied specious arguments to those who asserted, with the ingenious author of the Fable of the Bees,* that "private vices are public benefits;" and in consequence, its tendency appears to me essentially aristocratic and *demoralizing*, as tending to produce supine contentment with a vicious and degrading order of things. But Malthus himself declares the only proper check to be, the general practice of celibacy to a late age. He employs all his eloquence to persuade men and women that they ought not to marry till they are twenty-eight or thirty; and that, if they do, they are contributing to the misery of the world.†

* Mandeville.
† Some wag, adverting to the fact, that Mr. Malthus himself has a large family, remarked, "that the reverend gentleman knew better how to preach than to practise."

Now, Mr. Malthus may preach for ever on this subject. Individuals may indeed be found, who will look to distant consequences, and sacrifice present enjoyment; even as individuals are found to become and remain Shaking Quakers: but to believe that the mass of mankind will **abjure,** through the ten fairest years of life, the nearest and dearest of social relations; and during the very holiday of existence, will live the life of monks and nuns— all to avert a catastrophe which is confessedly some hundreds of years distant—to believe this, requires a faith **which no** accurate observer of mankind possesses.

This weak point the aristocratic expounders of Malthus' **doctrines** were not slow to discover. They broadly **asserted, that** such "moral restraint" would never be generally practised. They asked, whether a young woman, to whom a comfortable home and a pleasant companion were offered, would refuse to accept them, on this theory of population; whether a young man who had a fair (or even but a very indifferent) prospect of maintaining a family, would doom himself to celibacy **lest the** world should be overpeopled. And they put it **to the** advocates of late marriages, whether, in one sex at least, the recommendation, if even nominally followed, would not almost certainly lead to vicious excess and degrading associations; thus resolving the check into vice and misery at last. If experience answered these questions in the negative, was it not clear, (they would exultingly ask,) that vice and misery are the natural lot of man; and that it is quixotic, if not impious, to plague ourselves about them, or to attempt, by their suppression, to controvert the decrees of God?

It was very easy for generous feelings to reply to so heartless an **argument.** It was easy to **ask,** whether even the apparent hopelessness of the case formed any legitimate **apology** for supine indifference ; or whether, where we cannot cure, we are absolved from the duty of alleviating. But it was not very easy fully and fairly to meet the question. It was idle to deny that preaching would not put off marriage for ten years : and if no other species of moral restraint than ten years Shakerism could be proposed, it did appear evident enough, that moral restraint would be by the mass neglected, and that the physical checks of vice and misery must come into play **at** last.

I pray my readers, then, distinctly to observe how the matter stands. Population, unrestrained, *must* increase beyond the possibility of the earth and its produce to support. At present it is restrained by vice and misery. The only remedy which the orthodoxy of the English clergyman permits him to propose, is, late marriages. The most enlightened observers of mankind are agreed, that nothing contributes **so positively** and immediately to demoralize a nation, as when its youth refrain, until a late period, from forming disinterested connexions with those of the other sex. The frightful increase of prostitutes, the destruction of health, the rapid spread of intemperance, the ruin of moral feelings, are, to the mass, the *certain* consequences. Individuals there are, who escape the contagion ; individuals whose better feelings revolt, under *any* temptation, from the mercenary embrace, or the Circean cup of intoxication; but these are exceptions only. The mass must have their pleasures; the pleasures of intellectual intercourse, of unbought affection, and of good taste and good feeling, if they can ; but if they cannot, **then such pleasures (alas** ! that language should be perverted to entitle them to the name !)

as the sacrifice of money and the ruin of body and mind can purchase.*

But this is not all. Not only is Malthus' proposition fraught with immorality, in that it discountenances to a late age those disinterested sexual connexions which can alone save youth from vice ; but it is *impracticable*. Men and women will scarcely pause to calculate the chances they have of affording support to their children ere they become parents: how, then, should they stop to calculate the chances of the world's being overpeopled? Malthus may say what he pleases, they never will make any such calculation ; and it is folly to expect they **should**.

Let us observe, then : *unless some less ascetic and more practicable species of "moral restraint" be introduced,* vice and misery will *ultimately* become the inevitable lot of man upon earth. He can no more escape them, than he can the light of the sun, or the stroke of death.

What an incitement, this, to the prosecution of our enquiry! Here is a principle set up, which is all but an **apology** for the apathy that prevails among the rich and **the** powerful—among governors and legislators—in regard to human improvement. How important, how essential for the interests of virtue, that it should be refuted ! How beneficent that knowledge, which discloses to us some moral, practicable check to population, and relieves us from the despairing conclusion, that the irrevocable doom of man is misery, without remedy and without end ! In the absence of such knowledge, truly the prospects of the world were dark and cheerless. The modern

---

* Lawrence, the ingenious author of the " Empire of the Nairs," says shrewdly enough, " Wherever the women are prudes, the men will be drunkards."

doctrine of population has weighed like a spell on the exertions of benevolence, and chilled, almost to inaction, even the warm heart of charity. Philanthropy herself pauses, **when** she begins **to fear that all her exertions** are to result in hopeless disappointment. And yet— such is this world—even the ablest opponents of Malthus stop short when they come to the question, and leave an argument unanswered, which a dozen pages might suffice for ever to set at rest.

Let one of the most intelligent of these opponents, a man of splendid and sterling talent—let MILL, the celebrated political economist and talented author of "British India," speak for himself.

I extract from the article "Colony," in the supplement to the Encyclopædia Britannica, and which is from **the** pen of Mill, the following paragraph:

"**What are the** best means of checking the progress of population, **when it cannot go** on unrestrained without producing one or other of two most undesirable effects, either drawing an undue portion of the population to the mere raising of food, or producing poverty and wretchedness, it is not now the time to enquire. *It is, indeed, the most important practical problem to which the wisdom of the politician and the moralist can be applied.* It has, till this time, been miserably evaded by all those who have meddled with the subject, as well as by those who were called upon by their situation to find a remedy for the evils to which it relates. And yet, *if the superstitions of the nursery were disregarded, and the principle of utility kept steadily in view,* a solution might not be very difficult to be found; and the means of drying up one of the most copious sources of human **evil—a** source which *if all other sources were taken* *away, might alone suffice to retain the great mass of human beings in misery*, might be seen to be neither doubtful nor difficult to be applied."

Let my readers bear in mind, that this is from the pen of one of the most justly admired writers of the present day; a man celebrated throughout all Europe, for his works on political economy, and whose writings are not unknown even on this side the Atlantic. He considers the question now under discussion to involve " the most important problem to which the wisdom of the politician and moralist can be applied." This question, he admits, **has ever been " miserably** evaded." Yet even a man so influential and enlightened as Mill, must himself yield to the weakness he reprobates ; must speak in parables, as the Nazarene reformer did before him ; and, even while commenting on the " miserable evasion" of a subject so engrossingly important, must imitate the very evasion he despises.

I will not imitate it. I am more independently situa**ted** than the English economist ; and I see, as clearly as he does, the extreme importance of the subject. What he saw and declared *ought* to be said, I will say.

Before concluding this chapter, let me state distinctly, that I by no means agree with Malthus and other political economists in believing, that, at this moment, there is an actual excess of population in any country (China perhaps excepted) in the known world. I believe that there is more than enough land in every country of Europe to support, in perfect comfort, all its present **inhabitants.** That they *are* not supported in comfort, **is, in my** opinion, attributable, not to overpopulation, but to mal-government. Monopolies favour the rich, taxes oppress the poor, commercial rivalry grinds its victims to the dust. To such causes as these, **and not to over-population,** *at the time being,* is the mass of distress (felt more or less over the civilized **world) to be attributed. Thus, if the enemies of reform would but let us alone,** we might long postpone to other and more **important** discussions, this population question. But they **will not.** They *force* it upon us. And though **it might have evinced want of** judgment to obtrude it **unnecessarily or prematurely** on the public, it would **betray cowardice to evade it now, when thrust upon us.**

Besides, though it be undeniable that iniquitous **laws and a vicious order of things often produce the result** that is falsely attributed to overpopulation, **it is yet equally undeniable, that the most perfect system of laws in** the world could not *ultimately* prevent **the evils of a** superabundant **population. And it is no less certain, that, in the meantime, the pressure of a large family on the labouring man greatly augments the evil, and often deprives him of that very leisure which he might employ in devising constitutional means to better his condition, instead of leaving public** business **in the hands of** political **gamblers. Thus an** answer **to the population question is offered as an** *alleviation* **of** existing evils, **not as a** *cure* **for** them. Population **might be** but half what **it is, and unjust** legislation **and vicious** customs **would still give birth, as they now do, to luxury and want. The laws and customs ought to be,** *must* **be changed; but, while the grass is growing, let us prevent the horse from starving, if we can.**

Enough has been said, probably, in this chapter, to determine the question, whether it is, or is not, *desirable,* in a political point of view, that some check to population be sought and disclosed—some " moral restraint" that shall not, like vice and misery, be demoralizing, nor, like late marriages, be ascetic and impracticable.

CHAPTER V.

THE QUESTION CONSIDERED IN ITS SOCIAL BEARINGS.

This is by far the most important branch of the question. The evils caused by an overstocking of the world, if even inevitable, are distant; and an abstract view of the subject, however unanswerable, does **not** come home to the mind with the force of detailed reality.

What would be the probable effect, in social life, if mankind obtained and exercised a control over the instinct of reproduction?

My settled conviction is—and I am prepared to defend it—that the effect would be salutary, moral, civilizing; that it would prevent many crimes and more unhappiness; that it would lessen intemperance and profligacy; that it would polish the manners and improve the moral feelings; that it would relieve the burden of the poor, and the cares of the rich; that it would most essentially benefit the rising generation, by enabling parents generally more carefully to educate, and more comfortably to provide for, their offspring. I proceed to substantiate as I may these positions.

And first, let us look solely to the situation of married persons. Is it not notorious, that the families of the married often increase beyond what a regard for the young beings coming into the world, or the happiness **of those who give them birth, would dictate?** In how many instances does the hard-working father, and more especially the mother, of a poor family, remain slaves throughout their lives, tugging at the oar of incessant labour, toiling to live, and living only to die ; when, if their offspring had been limited to two or three only, they might have enjoyed comfort and comparative affluence ! **How often is the health of the mother, giving birth every year to an infant**—happy, if it be **not twins** !—and compelled to toil on, even at those times when nature imperiously calls for some relief from daily drudgery—how often is the mother's comfort, health, nay, her life, thus sacrificed ! **Or, if care and toil have weighed down the spirit, and at last broken the health of the father, how often is the widow left, unable, with the most virtuous intentions, to save her fatherless** offspring from **becoming degraded** objects of **charity,** or profligate votaries of vice !

Fathers and mothers ! **not you who have your nursery and your nursery maids,** and who leave your children **at home, to frequent the** crowded rout, or to glitter in the hot ball-room ; but you by the labour of whose hands **your children** are to live, and who, as you count their rising numbers, sigh to think how soon sickness or misfortune may lessen those wages which are now **but just** sufficient to afford them bread—fathers **and mothers in humble life !** to you my argument comes home, with the **force of reality. Others may impugn—may ridicule it. By bitter experience you know and feel its truth.**

It will be said, that government ought to provide for the **support and education of all the** children of the land. **No one is less inclined to deny** the position **than I. But it** *does* not **support and educate** them. **And, if it did, a period must come at last, when even such an act** of justice would be no relief from the evils of over-population.

Yet this is not all. Every physician knows, that there are many women so constituted that they cannot give birth to healthy—sometimes not to *living* children. Is it desirable—is it *moral*, that such women should become pregnant? Yet this is continually the case, the warnings of physicians to the contrary notwithstanding. Others there are, who ought never to become parents; because, **if they do, it is only to transmit to their** offspring grievous hereditary diseases; perhaps that worst of diseases, insanity. Yet they will not lead a life of celibacy. They marry. They become parents, **and** the world **suffers by it. That a human** being should give birth to a child, knowing that he transmits to it hereditary disease, is, in my opinion, an immorality. But it is a folly to expect that we can ever induce all such **persons to** live the lives of Shakers. Nor is it necessary: all that duty requires of them is, to refrain from becoming parents. Who can estimate the beneficial effect which rational moral restraint may thus have, on **the health,** beauty, and physical improvement of our **race, throughout future generations!**

But, apart from these latter considerations, is it not most plainly, clearly, incontrovertibly *desirable*, that parents *should have the power** to limit their offspring, whether they choose to exercise it or not? Who *can* lose by their having this power? and how many *may* gain!

---

* It may perhaps be argued, that all married persons *have* this power already, seeing that they are no more obliged to become parents than the unmarried; they may live as the brethren and sisters among the Shakers do. But this Shaker remedy is, in the first place, utterly impracticable, as a general rule; and, secondly, it would chill and embitter domestic life, even if it were practicable.

may gain competency for themselves, and the opportunity carefully to educate and provide for their children! How many may escape the jarrings, the quarrels, the disorder, the anxiety, which an overgrown family too often causes in the domestic circle!

It sometimes happens, that individual instances come home to the feelings with greater force than any general reasoning. I shall, in this place, adduce one which came immediately under my cognizance.

In June, 1829, I received from an elderly gentleman of the first respectability, occupying a public situation in one of the western states, a letter, requesting to know whether I could afford any information or advice in a case which greatly interested him, and which regarded a young woman for whom he had ever experienced the sentiments of a father. In explanation of the circumstances to which he alluded, he enclosed me a copy of a letter which she had just written to him, and which I here transcribe verbatim. A letter more touching from its simplicity, or more strikingly illustrative of the unfortunate situation in which not one, but thousands, in married life, find themselves placed, I have never read.

L***, Kentucky, May 3, 1829.

Dear Sir,

The friendship which has existed between you and my father, ever since I can remember; the unaffected kindness you used to express towards me, when you resided in our neighbourhood, during my childhood; the lively solicitude you have always seemed to feel for my welfare, and your benevolent and liberal character, induce me to lay before you, in a few words, my critical situation, and ask you for your kind advice.

It is my lot to be united in wedlock to a young mechanic of industrious habits, good dispositions, pleasing manners, and agreeable features, excessively fond of our children and of me; in short, eminently well qualified to render himself and family and all around him happy, were it not **for the** besetting sin of drunkenness. About once in every three or four weeks, if he meet, either accidentally or purposely, with some of his friends, of whom, either real or pretended, his good nature and liberality procure him many, he is sure to get intoxicated, so as to lose his reason; and, when thus beside **himself, he** trades and makes foolish bargains, so much to his disadvantage, that he has almost reduced himself and family to beggary, being no longer able to keep a shop of his own, but obliged to work journey work.

We have not been married quite four years, and have already given being to three dear little ones. Under present circumstances, what can I expect will be their fate and mine? I shudder at the prospect before me. With my excellent constitution and industry, and the labour of my husband, I feel able to bring up these three little cherubs in decency, were I to have no more: but when I seriously consider my situation, I can see no other al**ternative left for me, than to tear myself away from the man who,** though addicted to **occasional intoxication,** would sacrifice his life for my sake; **and for whom,** contrary to my father's will, I successively refused **the hand** and wealth of a lawyer and of a preacher; or continue to witness his degradation, and bring into existence, in **all p**robability, a numerous family of helpless and desti**tute children,** who, on account of poverty, must inevita**bly be doomed to a** life of ignorance, and consequent **vice and misery.**

The dreadful sentence pronounced against me by my father for my disobedience, forbids **me** applying to him, either for advice or any thing else. My husband being somewhat sceptical, my father **attributes his intemperance** to his infidelity; though my brother, as you know, being a member of the same church with my father, is nevertheless, though he does not fool away his property, more of a drunkard than my husband, and ranks among the faithful. You will therefore plainly see, that for these and other reasons, I stand the more in need of your friendly advice; and I do hope and believe, you **will** give me such advice and counsel as you would **to your** own daughter, had you one in the same predicament that I am. In so doing, you will add new claims to the gratitude of your friend, **M. W.**

Need I add **one word** of comment on such a case as this? Every feeling mind must be touched by the amiable feeling and good sense that pervade the **letter. Every** rational being, surely, must admit, that the power of preventing, without injury or sacrifice, the increase of a family, under such circumstances, is a public benefit and a private blessing.

Will it be asserted—and I know no other even plausible reply to these facts and arguments—will it be asserted, that the thing is, in itself, immoral or unseemly? I deny it; and I point to the population of France, in justification of my denial. Where will you **find, on the face of** the globe, a more polished or **more civilized nation** than the French, or one **more punctiliously alive to any** rudeness, coarseness, or indecorum? You will find none. The French are **scrupulous on these points, to a proverb. Yet,** as every intelligent traveller in France must have **remarked,** there is scarcely to be found, among the middle or upper classes, (and seldom even among **the working classes,) such a** thing **as a large** family;

very seldom more than three or four children. A French lady of the utmost delicacy and respectability will, in common conversation, say as simply—(ay, and as *innocently*, whatever the self-righteous prude may aver to the contrary)—as she would proffer any common remark about the weather: " I have three children; my husband and I think that is as many as we can do justice to, and I do not intend to have any more."*

I have stated notorious facts, facts which no traveller who has visited Paris, and seen any thing of the domestic life of its inhabitants, will attempt to deny. However heterodox, then, my view of the subject may be in this country, I am supported in it by the opinion and the practice of the most refined and most socially cultivated nation in the world.

Will it still be argued, that the practice, if not coarse, is immoral? Again I appeal to France. I appeal to the details of the late glorious revolution—to the innumerable instances of moderation, of courage, of honesty, of disinterestedness, of generosity, of magnanimity, displayed on the memorable "three days," and ever since; and I challenge comparison between the national character of France for virtue, as well as politeness, and that of any other nation under heaven.

It is evident, then, that, to married persons, the power of limiting their offspring to their circumstances is most desirable. It may often promote the harmony, peace, and comfort of families; sometimes it may save from bankruptcy and ruin, and sometimes it may rescue the mother from premature death. In *no* case can it, by

* Will our sensitive fine ladies blush at the plain good sense and simplicity of such an observation? Let me tell them, the indelicacy is in their own minds, not in the words of the French mother.

possibility, be worse than superfluous. *In no case can it be mischievous.*

If the moral feelings were carefully cultivated, if we were taught to consult, in every thing, rather the welfare of those we love than our own, how strongly would these arguments be felt! No man ought even to *desire* that a woman should become the mother of his children, unless it was her express wish, and unless he knew it to be for her welfare, that she should. Her feelings, her interests, should be for him in this matter *an imperative law.* She it is who bears the burden, and therefore with her also should the decision rest. Surely it may well be a question whether it be desirable, or whether any man ought to ask, that the whole life of an intellectual, cultivated woman, should be spent in bearing a family of twelve or fifteen children; to the ruin, perhaps, of her constitution, if not to the overstocking of the world. No man ought to require or expect it.

Shall I be told, that this is the very romance of morality? Alas! that what ought to be a matter of every day practice—a common-place exercise of the duties and charities of life—a bounden duty—an instance of domestic courtesy too universal either to excite remark or to merit commendation—alas! that a virtue so humble that its absence ought to be reproached as a crime, should, to our selfish perceptions, seem but a fastidious refinement, or a fanciful supererogation!

But I pass from the case of married persons to that of young men and women who have yet formed no matrimonial connexion.

In the present state of the world, when public opinion stamps with opprobrium every sexual connexion which has not received the orthodox sanction of an oath, almost all young persons, on reaching the age of maturity, desire to marry. The heart must be very cold, or very isolated, that does not find some object on which to bestow its affections. Thus, early marriages would be almost universal, did not prudential considerations interfere. The young man thinks, " I must not marry yet. I cannot support a family. I must make money first, and think of a matrimonial settlement afterwards."

And so he goes to making money, fully and sincerely resolved, in a few years, to share it with her whom he now loves. But passions are strong, and temptations great. Curiosity, perhaps, introduces him into the company of those poor creatures whom society first reduces to a dependence on the most miserable of mercenary trades, and then curses for being what she has made them. There his health and his moral feelings alike make shipwreck. The affections he had thought to treasure up for their first object, are chilled by dissipation and blunted by excess. He scarcely retains a passion but avarice. Years pass on—years of profligacy and speculation—and his first wish is accomplished; his fortune is made. Where now are the feelings and resolves of his youth?

> Like the dew on the mountain,
> **Like the foam on the river,**
> Like the bubble on the fountain,
> They are gone—and for ever!

He is a man of pleasure—a man of the world. **He** laughs at the romance of his youth, and marries a fortune. If gaudy equipages and gay parties confer happiness, he is happy. But if these be only the sunshine on the stormy ocean below, he is a victim to that system of morality, which forbids a reputable connexion until the period when provision has been made for a large, expected family. Had he married the first object of his choice, and simply delayed becoming a father until his prospects seemed to warrant it, how different might have been his lot! Until men and women are absolved from the fear of becoming parents, except when they themselves desire it, they ever will form mercenary and demoralizing connexions, and seek in dissipation the happiness they might have found in domestic life.

I know that this, however common, is not a universal case. Sometimes the heavy responsibilities of a family are incurred, at all risks; and who shall say how often a life of unremitting toil and poverty is the consequence? Sometimes—if even rarely—the young mind *does* hold to its first resolves. The youth plods through years of cold celibacy and solitary anxiety; happy, if before the best hours of life are gone, and its warmest feelings withered, he may return to claim the reward of his forbearance and his industry. But even in this comparatively happy case, shall we count for nothing the years of ascetical sacrifice at which after-happiness is purchased? The days of youth are not too many, nor its affections too lasting. We may, indeed, if a great object require it, sacrifice the one and mortify the other. But is this, in itself, desirable? Does not wisdom tell us, that such sacrifice is a dead loss—to the warm-hearted often a grievous one? Does not wisdom bid us temperately enjoy the spring-time of life, " while the evil days come not, nor the years draw nigh, when we shall say, ' We have no pleasure in them?' "

Let us say, then, if we will, that the youth who thus sacrifices the present for the future, chooses wisely between two evils, profligacy and asceticism. This is true. But let us not imagine the lesser evil to be a good. It is *not* good for man to be alone. It is for no man's or woman's happiness or benefit, that they should be condemned to Shakerism. It is a violence done to the feelings, and an injury to the character. A life of rigid celibacy, though infinitely preferable to a life of dissipation, is yet fraught with many evils. Peevishness, restlessness, vague longings, and instability of character, are among the least of these. The mind is unsettled, and the judgment warped. Even the very instinct which is thus mortified, assumes an undue importance, and occupies a portion of the thoughts which does not of right or nature belong to it; and which, during a life of satisfied affection, it would not obtain.

I speak not now of extreme cases, where solitary vice* or disease, or even insanity, has been the result of ascetical mortification. I speak of every day cases; and I am well convinced, that, (however wise it often is, in the present state of the world, to select and adhere to this alternative,) yet no man or woman can live the life of a conscientious Shaker, without suffering, more or less, both physically, mentally, and morally. This is the more to be regretted, because the very noblest portion of

---

* For a vice so unnatural as onanism there could be no possible temptation, and therefore no existence, were not men unnaturally and mischievously situated. It first appeared, probably, in monasteries; and has been perpetuated by the more or less anti-social and demoralizing relation in which the sexes stand to each other, in almost all countries. In estimating the consequences of the present false situation of society, we must set down to the black account the wretched, wretched consequences (terminating not unfrequently in incurable insanity) of this vice, the preposterous offspring of modern civilization. Physicians say that onanism at present prevails, to a lamentable extent, both in this country and England. If the recommendations contained in this little treatise were generally followed, it would probably totally disappear in a single generation.

our species—the good, the pure, the high-minded, and the kind-hearted—are the chief victims.

Thus, inasmuch **as** the scruple of incurring heavy responsibilities deters from forming moral connexions, and encourages intemperance and prostitution, the knowledge which enables man to limit his offspring, would, in the present state of things, save much unhappiness and prevent many crimes. Young persons sincerely attached to each other, and who might wish to marry, would marry early; merely resolving not to become parents until prudence permitted it. The young man, instead of solitary toil or vulgar dissipation, would enjoy the society and the assistance of her he had chosen as his companion; and the best years of life, whose pleasures never return, **would not** be squandered **in riot, or lost** through **mortification.**

My readers will remark, **that** all the arguments **I have hitherto** employed, apply strictly to the present order of things, and the present laws and system of marriage. No one, therefore, need be a moral heretic on this subject to admit and approve them. The marriage laws might all remain for ever as they are; and yet a moral check to population would be beneficent and important.

But there are other cases, it will be said, where the **knowledge of such a check would be mischievous. If young women,** it will **be argued, were absolved from the fear of consequences, they would** rarely preserve their **chastity. Unlegalized** connexions **would** be common and seldom **detected.** Seduction would be facilitated. Let us dispassionately **examine** this argument.

I fully agree with that most amiable of moral heretics, **Shelley, that** " Seduction, which term could have no meaning in a rational society, has now a most tremendous one."* It matters not how artificial the penalty which society has chosen to affix to a breach of her capricious decrees. Society has the power in her own hands; and that moral Shylock, Public Opinion, enforces the penalty, even though it cost the life of the victim. The consequences, then, to the poor sufferer, whose offence is, at most, but an error of judgment or a weakness of the heart, are the same as if her imprudence were indeed a crime of the blackest dye. And his conduct who, for a momentary, selfish gratification, will deliberately entail a life of wretchedness on one whose chief fault, perhaps, was her misplaced confidence in a villain, is not one whit excused by the folly and injustice of the sentence.† Some poet says,

> "The man who lays his hand upon a woman
> Save in the way of kindness, is a wretch
> Whom 'twere gross flattery to call a coward."

What epithet, then, belongs to him who makes it a trade to win a woman's gentle affections, betray her generous confidence, and then, when the consequences become apparent, abandon her to dependence, and the scorn of a cold, a self-righteous, and a wicked world; a

---

* See letter of Percy Byssche Shelley, published in the "Lion," of December 5, 1828.

† Every reflecting mind will distinguish between the unreasoning—sometimes even generous, imprudence of youthful passion, and the calculating selfishness of the matured and heartless libertine. It is a melancholy truth, that pseudo-civilization produces thousands of seducers by profession, who, while daily calling the heavens to witness their eternal affections, have no affection for any thing on earth but their own precious and profligate selves. It is to characters so utterly worthless as these that my observations apply.

world which will forgive any thing but rebellion against its tyranny, and in whose eyes it seems the greatest of crimes to be unsuspecting and warm-hearted! I will give my hand freely to a galley-slave, and speak to the highway-robber as to an honest man; but there is one character with whom I desire to exchange neither word nor greeting—the cold-hearted, deliberate, practised, and calculating seducer!

And, let me ask, what is it gives to the arts of seduction their sting, and stamps to the world its victim? Why is it, that the man goes free and enters society again, almost courted and applauded for his treachery while the woman is a mark for the finger of reproach, and a butt for the tongue of scandal? Because she bears about her the mark of what is called her disgrace. She becomes a mother; **and society has something** tangible against which to direct its anathemas. **Nine** tenths, at **least, of the misery and** ruin which are caused **by seduction, even in the present state of** public opinion on **the** subject, result from cases of pregnancy. **Perhaps the** unfeeling **selfishness of him who fears to become a** father, administers some noxious drug to procure abortion; perhaps—for even such scenes our courts of justice disclose!—perhaps the frenzy of the wretched mother takes the life of her infant, or seeks in suicide the consummation of her **wrongs and** her woes! Or, if the little being lives, the **dove in** the falcon's claws **is not** more certain of death, **than we may be, that society will visit, with its bitterest scoffs and reproaches, the bruised** spirit of the mother and the unconscious innocence of the child.

If, then, we cannot **do** all, shall we neglect a part? **If we** cannot prevent every misery which man's selfishness and the world's cruelty entail **on a sex which it** ought to be our pride and honour to cherish and defend; let us prevent as many as we can. If we cannot persuade society to revoke its unmanly and *unchristian** persecution of those who are often the best and gentlest of its members—let us, at the least, give to woman what defence we may, against its violence.

I appeal to any father, trembling for the reputation of his child, whether, **if she were induced to form an un**legalized connexion, her pregnancy would not be a frightful aggravation? I appeal to him, whether any innocent preventive which shall save her from a situation that must soon disclose all to the world, would not be an act of mercy, of charity, of philanthropy—whether it might not save him from despair, and her from ruin? The fastidious conformist may frown upon the question, but to the father it comes home; and, whatever his lips may say, his heart will acknowledge the soundness and the force of the argument it conveys.†

---

* Jesus said unto her, " Neither do I condemn thee."—*John* viii. 11.

† What **is the** actual state of society in Great Britain, and even **in this republic,** that pseudo-civilization, in her superlative delicacy, should so fastidiously scruple to speak of or to sanction a simple, moral, effectual check to population? Are her sons all **chaste and temperate, and her** daughters all **passionless and** pure? I might disclose, if I would, in this very **city of** New-York—and in our neighbour city of Philadelphia—scenes and practices that have come to light from time to time, and that would furnish no very favourable answer to the question. I might ask, whether all the houses of assignation in these two cities are frequented by the known profligate alone? or, whether **some of the most outwardly respectable** fathers—ay, *mothers* **of families—have not been found in resorts supported and frequented** only by " good society" like themselves?

As regards Great Britain, **I** might quote the evidence delivered before a " Committee of the House of Commons, on Labourers'

It may be, that some sticklers for orthodox morality will still demur to the positions I defend. They will perhaps tell me, as the Committee of a certain Society in this city lately did, that the power of preventing conceptions "holds out inducements and facilities for the prostitution of their daughters, their sisters, and their wives."*

Wages," by Henry Drummond, a banker, magistrate, and large land-owner in the county of Surry, in which the following question and answer occur: Q. "What is the practice you allude to of forcing marriages?" A. "I believe nothing is more erroneous than the assertion, that the poor laws tend to imprudent marriages; I never knew an instance of a girl being married until she was with child, nor ever knew of a marriage taking place through a calculation for future support." Mr. Drummond's assertions were confirmed by other equally respectable witnesses; and from what I have myself learnt in conversation with some of the chief manufacturers of England, I am convinced, that the statement, as regards the working population in the chief manufacturing districts, is scarcely exaggerated.

I might go on to state, that the spot on which the Foundling Hospital in Dublin now stands, formerly went by the name of "Murderer's Lane," from the number of child murders that were perpetrated in the vicinity.

I might adduce the testimony of respectable witnesses in proof, that, even among the married, the blighting effects of ergot are not unfrequently incurred; by those very persons, probably, who, in public, would think fit to be terribly shocked at this little book.

But why multiply proofs? The records of every court of justice, nay, the tittle tattle of every fashionable drawing-room, sufficiently marks the real character of this prudish and pharisaical world of ours.

* See letter of the Committee of the Typographical Society to Robert Dale Owen, published in the Commercial Advertiser of the 29th of September, and copied into the Free Enquirer of the 9th of October, 1830.

For a statement of the circumstances connected with that letter, and which induced me, at this time, to write and publish the present treatise, see Preface.

Truly, but they pay their wives, their sisters, and their daughters, a poor compliment! Is, then, this vaunted chastity a mere thing of circumstance and occasion? Is there but the difference of opportunity between it and prostitution? Would their wives, and their sisters, and their daughters, if once absolved from the fear of offspring, all become prostitutes—all sell their embraces for gold, and descend to a level with the most degraded? In truth, but they slander their own kindred; they libel their own wives, sisters, and daughters. If they spoke truth—if fear were indeed the only safeguard of their relatives' chastity, little value should I place on a virtue like that! and small would I esteem his offence, who should attempt or seduce it.*

* I should like to hear these gentlemen explain, according to what principle they imagine the chastity of their *wives* to grow out of a fear of offspring; so that, if released from such fear, prostitution would follow. I can readily comprehend that the unmarried may be supposed careful to avoid that situation to which no legal cause can be assigned; but a wife must be especially dull, if she cannot assign, in all cases, a legal cause; and a husband must be especially sagacious, if he can tell whether the true cause be assigned or not. This safeguard to married chastity, therefore, to which the gentlemen of the Typographical Committee seem to look with so implicit a confidence, is a mere broken reed; and has been so, ever since the days of Bathsheba.

Yet *conjugal* chastity is that which is especially valued. The inconstancy of a wife commonly cuts much deeper than the dishonour of a sister. In that case, then, which the world usually considers of the highest importance, the fear of offspring *imposes no check whatever*. It cannot make one iota of difference whether a married woman be knowing in physiology or not; except perhaps, indeed, to the husband's advantage; in cases where the wife's conscience induces her at least to guard against the possibility of burthening her legal lord with the care and support of children that are not his. Constancy, where it actually exists, is the offspring of something more efficacious than ignorance

That chastity which is worth preserving is not the chastity that owes its birth to fear and to ignorance. If to enlighten a woman regarding a simple physiological fact will make her a prostitute, she must be especially predisposed to profligacy. But it is a libel on the sex. Few, indeed, there are, who would continue so miserable and degrading a calling, could they but escape from it. For one prostitute that is made by inclination, ten are made by necessity. Reform the laws—equalize the comforts of society, and you need withhold no knowledge from your wives and daughters. It is want, not knowledge, that leads to prostitution.

For myself, I would withhold from no sister, or daughter, or wife of mine, any ascertained fact whatever. It should be to me a duty and a pleasure to communicate to them all I knew myself: and I should hold it an insult to their understandings and their hearts to imagine, that their virtue would diminish as their knowledge increased. Vice is never the offspring of just knowledge; and they who say it is, slander their own nature. Would we but trust human nature, instead of continually suspecting it, and guarding it by bolts and bars, and thinking to make it very chaste by keeping it very ignorant, what a different world we should have of it!

And if in the wife's case, men must and do trust to something else, why not in all other cases, where restraint may be considered desirable? Shall men trust in the greater, and fear to trust in the less? Whatever any one may choose to assert regarding his relatives' secret inclinations to profligacy, these arguments may convince him, that if he has any safeguard at present, a perusal of Moral Physiology will not destroy it.

'Tis strange that men, by way of suborning an argument, should be willing thus to vilify their relatives' character and motives, without first carefully examining whether any thing was gained to their cause, after all, by the vilification.

The virtue of ignorance is a sickly plant, ever exposed to the caterpillar of corruption, liable to be scorched and blasted even by the free light of heaven; of precarious growth; and, even if at last artificially matured, of little or no real value.

I know that parents often think it right and proper to withhold from their children—especially from their daughters—facts the most influential on their future lives, and the knowledge of which is essential to every man and woman's well-being.* Such a course has ever appeared to me ill-judged and productive of very injurious effects. A girl is surely no whit the better for believing, until her marriage night, that children are found among the cabbage leaves in the garden. The imagination is excited, the curiosity kept continually on the stretch; and that which, if simply explained, would have been recollected only as any other physiological phenomenon, assumes all the rank and importance and engrossing interest of a mystery. Nay, I am well convinced, that mere curiosity has often led ignorant young people into situations, from which a little more confidence and openness on the part of their parents or guardians, would have effectually secured them.

In the monkish days of mental darkness, when it was taught and believed, that all the imaginations and all the

---

* Instances innumerable might be adduced. Not one young person, for example, in twenty, is ever told, that sexual intercourse during the period of a woman's courses is not unfrequently productive, to the woman of a species of fluor albus, and sometimes (as a consequent) to the man of symptoms very similar to those of syphilis, but more easily removed. Yet what fact more important to be communicated? And how ridiculous the mischievously prudish refinement that conceals from human beings what it most deeply concerns them to know?

thoughts of man are only evil continually—when it was deemed right and proper to secure the submission of the mass by withholding from them the knowledge even how to read and write—in those days, it was all very well to **shut up** the physiological page, and tell us, that on the day we read therein we should surely die. But those times are past. In this nineteenth century, men and women read, think, discuss, enquire, judge for themselves. If, in these latter days, there is to be **virtue at all**, she must be the offspring of knowledge and of free **enquiry,** not of ignorance and mystery. We *cannot* prevent the spread of any real knowledge, even if we would; we *ought* not, even if we could.

This book will make its way through the whole United States. Curiosity and the notoriety which has already been given to the subject, will suffice at first to obtain for it circulation. The practical importance of the subject it treats will do the rest. It needed but some one to start the stone; its own momentum will suffice to carry it forward.

But, if we *could* prevent the circulation of truth, why *should* we? **We are not** afraid of it ourselves. No man thinks *his* morality will suffer by it. Each feels certain that his virtue can stand any degree of knowledge. And is it not the height of egregious presumption in each to imagine that his neighbour is so much weaker than himself, and requires a bandage which he can do **without?** Most of all, is it presumptuous to suppose, that that knowledge which the man of the world can bear with impunity, will corrupt the young and the **pure-hearted. It is the sullied** conscience only that suggests such fears. Trust youth and innocence. Speak to them openly. Show them that you respect **them, by** treating them with confidence; and they will quickly learn to respect and to govern themselves. You enlist even their pride in your behalf; and you will soon see them make it their boast and their highest pleasure to *merit* your confidence. But watch them, and show your suspicion of them but once—and you are the jailor, who will keep his prisoners just as long as bars and bolts shall prevent their escape. The world was never made for a prison-house; it is too large and ill-guarded: nor were parents ever intended for goal-keepers; their very affections unfit them for the task.

There is no more beautiful sight upon earth, than a family among whom there are no secrets and no reserves; where the young people confide every thing to their elder friends—for such to them are their parents—and where the parents trust every thing to their children; where each thought is communicated as freely as it arises; and all knowledge given, as simply as it is received. If the world contain a prototype of that Paradise, where nature is said to have known no sin or impropriety, it is such a family. And if there be a serpent that can poison the innocence of its inmates, that serpent is SUSPICION.

I ask no greater pleasure than thus to be the guardian and companion of young beings whose innocence shall speak to me as unreservedly as it thinks to itself; of young beings who shall never imagine that there is guilt in their thoughts, or sin in their confidence; and to whom, in return, I may impart every important and useful fact that is known to myself. Their virtue shall be of that hardy growth, which *all* facts tend to nourish and strengthen.

I put it to my readers, whether such a view of human nature, and such a mode of treating it, be not in accordance with the noblest feelings of their hearts. I put it to them, whether they have not felt themselves encouraged, improved, strengthened in every virtuous resolution, when they were generously trusted; and whether they have not felt abased and degraded, when they **were** suspiciously watched, and spied after, and kept in ignorance. If they find such feelings in their own hearts, let them not self-righteously imagine, that they only can be won by generosity, or that the nature of their fellow-creatures is different from their own.

There are other considerations connected with **this** subject, which farther attest the social advantages of the control I advocate. Human affections are **mutable, and** the sincerest of mortal resolutions may change.* Every day furnishes instances of alienations, and of separations; sometimes almost before the honey-moon is well expired. In such cases of unsuitability, it cannot be considered desirable that there should be offspring; and the power of refraining from becoming parents until intimacy had, in a measure, established the likelihood of permanent harmony of views and feelings, must be confessed to be advantageous.

The limits which my numerous avocations prescribe to this little treatise, permit me not to meet every argument in detail, which ingenuity or prejudice might put forward. If the world were not actually afraid to think freely or to listen to the suggestions of **common sense,** three fourths of **what has already been said would be** superfluous; for most of the arguments employed would

---

* Le premier serment que se firent deux êtres de chair, ce fut au pied d'un rocher, qui tombait en poussière; ils attestèrent de leur constance un ciel qui n'est pas un instant le même: tout passait en eux, et autour d'eux; et ils croyaient leurs cœurs affran**chis de** vicissitudes. O enfans! toujours enfans!

DIDEROT; *Jacques et son maitre.*

occur spontaneously to any rational, reasoning being. But the mass of mankind have still, in a measure, every thing to learn on this subject. The world seems to me much to resemble a company of gourmands, who sit down to a plentiful repast, first very punctiliously saying grace over it; and then, under sanction of the priest's blessing, think to gorge themselves with impunity; as conceiving, that gluttony after grace is no sin. So it is **with** popular customs and popular morality. Every thing is permitted, if external forms be but respected. Legal roguery is no crime, and ceremony-sanctioned excess no profligacy. The substance is sacrificed to the form, the virtue to the outward observance. The world troubles its head little about whether a man be honest or dishonest, so he knows how to avoid the penitentiary and escape the hangman. In like manner, the world seldom thinks it worth while to enquire whether a man be temperate or intemperate, prudent or thoughtless. It takes especial care to inform itself whether in all things he conforms to orthodox requirements; and, if he does, **all is right.** Thus men too often learn to consider an oath an absolution from all subsequent decencies and duties, and a full release from all after responsibilities. If a husband maltreat his wife, the offence is venal; for he premised it by making her, **at the altar, an** "honest woman." If a married father neglect his children, it is a trifle; for grace was regularly said, before they **were** born.

So **true is** this, that if some heterodox moralist were to throw out the idea, that many of the rudenesses and jarrings, and much **of the indifference and carelessness of each others' feelings that is exhibited in married** life, **might be traced to the** almost universal **custom (in** this country, though not **in France) of man and wife** continually occupying the same bed—if he put it to us whether such a forced and too frequent familiarity were not calculated to lessen the charms and pleasures, and diminish the respectful regard and deference, which ought ever to characterize the intercourse of human beings—if, I say, some heretical preferrer of things to forms were to light upon and express some such unlucky idea as this, ten to one the married portion of the community would fall upon him without mercy, as an impertinent intermeddler in their most legitimate rights and prerogatives.

With such a world as this, it is a difficult matter to reason. After listening to all I have said, it may perhaps cut me short by reminding me, that nature herself declares it to be right and proper, that we should reproduce our species without calculation or restraint. I will ask, in reply, whether nature also declares it to be right and proper, that, when the thermometer is at 96, we should drink greedily of cold water, and drop down dead in the streets? Let the world be told, that if nature gave us our passions and propensities, she gave us also the power wisely to control them; and that, when we hesitate to exercise that power, we descend to a level with the brute creation, and become the sport of fortune—the mere slaves of circumstance.*

* Some German poet, whose name has escaped me, says,

"Tapfer ist der Löwensieger,
Tapfer is der Weltbezwinger,
Tapferer, wer sich selbst bezwang!"

"Brave is the lion-victor,
Brave the conqueror of a world,
Braver, he who controls himself!"

It is a noble sentiment, and very appropriate to the present discussion.

To one other argument it were not, perhaps, worth while to advert, but that it has been already speciously used to excite popular prejudice. It has been said, that to recommend to mankind prudential restraint in cases where children cannot be provided for, is an insult to the poor man; since all ought to be so circumstanced that they might provide amply for the largest family. Most assuredly all *ought* to be so circumstanced; but all *are* not. And there would be just as much propriety in bidding a poor man go and take by force a piece of Saxony broadcloth from his neighbour's store, because he *ought* to be able to purchase it, as to encourage him to go on producing children, because he *ought* to have wherewithal to support them. Let us exert every nerve to correct the injustice and arrest the misery that results from a vicious order of things; but, until we have done so, let us not, for humanity's sake, madly recommend that which grievously aggravates the evil; which increases the burden on the present generation, and threatens with neglect and ignorance the next.

And now, let my readers pause. Let them review the various arguments I have placed before them. Let them reflect how intimately the instinct of which I treat is connected with the social welfare of society. Let them bear in mind, that just in proportion to its social influence, is it important that we should know how to control and govern it; that, when we obtain such control, we may save ourselves—and, what we ought to prize much more highly, may save our companions and our offspring, from suffering or misery; that, by such knowledge, the young may form virtuous connexions, instead of becoming profligates or ascetics; that, by it, early marriage is deprived of its heaviest consequences, and seduction of its sharpest sting; that, by it, man may be saved from moral ruin, and woman from desolating dishonour; that by it the first pure affections may be soothed and satisfied, instead of being thwarted or destroyed—let them call to mind all this, and then let them say, whether the possession of such control be not **a blessing to man.**

CHAPTER VI.

THE SUBJECT CONSIDERED IN ITS IMMEDIATE **CONNEXION WITH** PHYSIOLOGY.

It now remains, after having spoken of the *desirability* of obtaining control over the instinct of reproduction, to speak of its *practicability*.

As, in this world, the value of labour is too often estimated almost in proportion to its inutility, so, in physical science, contested questions seem to have attracted attention and engaged research, almost in the inverse ratio of their practical importance. We have a hundred learned hypotheses for one decisive practical experiment. We **have many** thousands of volumes written to explain fanciful theories, and **scarcely** as many dozens **to** record ascertained facts.

It **is not my** intention, **in** discussing this branch of the subject, **to examine the** hundred ingenious **theories** of generation which ancient and modern physiologists have **put forth.** I shall **not** enquire whether the future human being owes its first existence, as Hippocrates and Galen asserted, and Buffon very ingeniously supports, to the union of two life-giving fluids, **each a sort of extract of the body of the parent, and** composed **of** organic particles similar to the future offspring; or whether, as Harvey and Haller teach, the embryo reposes in the ovum until vivified by the seminal fluid, or perhaps only by the *aura seminalis;* or whether, according to the theories of Leuvenhoeck and Boerhaave, the future man first exists as a spermatic animalcula, for which the ovum becomes merely the nourishing receptacle; or whether, as the ingenious Andry imagines, a vivifying worm be the more correct hypothesis; or whether, finally, as Pérault will have it,* the embryo beings (too wonderfully organized to be supposed the production of any mere physical phenomenon) must be imagined to come directly from the hands of the Creator, who has filled the universe with these little germs, too minute, indeed, to exercise all the animal functions, but still self-existent, and awaiting only the insinuation of some subtle essence into their microscopic pores, to come forth as human beings. **Still less am** I inclined to follow Hippocrates and Tertullian in their enquiries, whether the soul is merely introduced into the fœtus, or pre-exists in the semen, and becomes, as it were, the architect of its future residence, the body;† or to attempt a refutation of the hypothesis of the metaphysical naturalist,‡ who asserts, (and adduces the infinite indivisibility of matter in support of the assertion,) that the actual germs of the whole human race, and of all that are yet **to be born, existed in the ovaria** of our first mother, **Eve. I leave these and fifty other** hypotheses as ingenious and as useless, **to be discussed by**

---

* See "Histoire de l'Académie des Sciences," for the year 1679, page 279.

† Hippocrates positively asserts this latter hypothesis, and is outrageous against all sceptics in his theory. In his work on diet, he tells us, " *Si quis non credat animam animæ misceri, demens est.*" Tertullian warmly supports the orthodoxy of this opinion.

‡ Bonner, I believe.

those who seem to make it a point of honour to leave no fact unexplained by some imagined theory; and I descend at once to the *terra firma* of positive experience and actual observation.

It is exceedingly to be regretted that mankind did not spend some small portion, at least, of the time and industry which has been wasted on theoretical researches, in collecting and collating the *actual experience* of human beings. But this task, too difficult for the ignorant, has generally been thought too simple and commonplace for the learned. To this circumstance, joined to the fact, that it is not thought fitting or decent for human beings freely **to communicate** their personal experience on the important subject now under consideration—to these causes are attributable the great and otherwise unaccountable ignorance which so strangely prevails, even sometimes among medical men, as to the power which man may possess over the reproductive instinct. Many physicians will positively **deny** that man possesses any such power. And yet, if **the** thousandth **part of the talent and research had been** employed to **investigate this** momentous fact, which has been turned to the building **up of idle theories,** no commonly intelligent **individual could well be ignorant** of the truth.

I have taken great pains to ascertain the opinions of the most enlightened physicians of Great Britain and France on this subject; (opinions which popular prejudice will not permit them to offer publicly in their works,) and they all concur in admitting, what the experience of the French nation *positively proves*, that man may have a perfect control over this instinct; and that men and women may, without any injury to health, or the slightest violence done to the moral feelings, and with but small diminution of the pleasure which accompanies

MORAL PHYSIOLOGY. 61

the gratification of the instinct, refrain at will from becoming parents. It has chanced to me, also, to win the confidence of several individuals, who have communicated to me, without reserve, their own experience; and all this has been corroborative of the same opinion.

Thus, though I pretend not to speak positively to the details of a subject, which will then only be fully understood when men acquire sense enough simply and unreservedly to discuss it, I may venture to assure my readers, that the main fact is incontrovertible. I shall adduce such facts in proof of this as may occur to me in the course of this investigation.

However various and contradictory the different theories of generation, almost all physiologists are agreed, that the entrance of the sperm itself (or of some volatile particles proceeding from it) into the uterus, must precede conception. This it was that probably first suggested the possibility of preventing conception at will.

Among the modes of preventing conception which may have prevailed in various countries, that which has been adopted, and is now universally practised, by the cultivated classes on the continent of Europe, by the French, the Italians, and, I believe, by the Germans and Spaniards, consists of complete withdrawal, on the part of the man, immediately previous to emission. *This is*, *in all cases*, *effectual.* It may be objected, that the practice requires a mental effort and a partial sacrifice. I reply, that, in France, where men consider this, (as it ought ever to be considered, when the interests of the other sex require it,) a *point of honour*—all young men learn to make the necessary effort; and custom renders it easy and a matter of course. As for the sacrifice, shall a trifling (and it is but a very trifling) diminution of physical enjoy-

6

ment be suffered to outweigh the most important considerations connected with the permanent welfare of those who are the nearest and dearest to us? Shall it be suffered to outweigh the risk of incurring heavy and sacred responsibilities, ere we are prepared to meet and fulfil them? Shall it be suffered to outweigh a regard for the comfort, the well-being—in some cases the *life*, of those whom we profess to love? The most selfish will hesitate deliberately to reply, in the affirmative, to such questions as these. A cultivated young Frenchman, instructed as he is, even from his infancy, carefully to consult, on all occasions, the wishes, and punctiliously to care for the comfort and welfare, of the gentler sex, would learn almost with incredulity, that, in other countries, there are men to be found, pretending to cultivation, who were less scrupulously honourable on this point than himself. You could not offer him a greater insult than to presuppose the possibility of his forgetting himself so far, as thus to put his own momentary gratification, for an instant, in competition with the wish or the well-being of any one to whom he professed regard or affection.*

I know it will be argued, that men in the mass are

---

* A Frenchman belonging to the cultivated classes, would as soon bear to be called a coward, as to be accused of causing the pregnancy of a woman, who did not desire it; and that, too, whether the matrimonial law had given him legal rights over her person or not. Such an imputation, if substantiated, would shut him out for ever from all decent society; and most properly so. It is a perfect barbarity, and ought to be treated as such.

When we begin to look to genuine morality, instead of empty or offensive forms, these are the principles of honour we shall implant in our children's minds: and then we shall have a world of courtesy and kindness, instead of a scene of legal outrage, or hypocritical profession not sufficiently moral to adopt this recommendation; because they will not make any voluntary sacrifice of animal enjoyment, however trifling. I do not see that. Hundreds of voluntary sacrifices are daily made to fashion—to public opinion. Let but public opinion bear on this point in other countries, as it does among the more enlightened classes in France, and similar effects will be produced.

Besides, the matter is a trifle. The mere act of **animal satisfaction**, counts with any man of commonly cultivated feelings, as but a small item in the aggregate of enjoyment which satisfied affection affords; **and, surely,** whether that act be at all times attended with the utmost degree of physical pleasure or not, must, even with the selfish, be a secondary and unimportant consideration. His moral sentiments must be especially weak or uncultivated, who will not admit, that it is the gratification of the social feelings—the repose of the affections—which at all times, constitutes the chief charm of human intercourse.

The least injurious among the present checks to population, celibacy, is a mortification of the affections, a violence done to the social feelings, sometimes a sacrifice even of the health. Not one of these objections **can be** urged to the trifling restraint proposed.

As to the cry which prejudice may raise **against it as** being unnatural, it is just as unnatural (and no **more so) as to refrain, in a** sultry **summer's day, from drinking, perhaps,** more than **a pint** of water at a draught, which prudence tells us is enough, while inclination would bid us drink **a quart.** *All* thwarting of any human wish **or** impulse may, **in** one sense, be called unnatural; it is not, however, ofttimes the less prudent and proper, on **that account.**

As to the practical efficacy of this simple preventive, the experience of France, where it is universally practised, might suffice in proof. I know, at this moment, several married persons who have told me, that, after having had as many children as they thought prudent, *they had for years employed this check, with perfect success.* For the satisfaction of my readers, I will select one particular instance.

I knew personally and intimately for many years a young man of strict honour, in whose sincerity I ever placed perfect confidence, and who confided to me the particulars of his situation. He was just entering on life, with slender means, and his circumstances forbade him to have a large family of children. He, therefore, having consulted with his young wife, practised this restraint, I believe for about eighteen months, and with perfect success. At the expiration of that period, their situation being more favourable, they resolved to become parents; and, in a fortnight after, the wife found herself pregnant. My friend told me, that though he felt the partial privation a little at first, a few weeks' habit perfectly reconciled him to it; and that nothing but a deliberate conviction that he might prudently now become a parent, and a strong desire on his wife's part to have a child, induced him to alter his first practice. I believe I was the only one among his friends to whom he ever communicated the real state of the case; and I doubt not there are, even in this country, hundreds of similar cases which the world never learns any thing about. Hence the doubts and ignorance which exist on the subject.

I add another instance. A few weeks since, a respectable and very intelligent father of a family, about thirty-five years of age, who resides west of the mountains, called at our office. Conversation turned on the present subject, and I expressed to him my conviction, that this check was effectual. He told me he could speak from personal experience. He had married young, and soon had three children. These he could support in comfort, without running into debt or difficulty; but, the price of produce sinking in his neighbourhood, there did not appear a fair prospect of supporting a large family. In consequence, he and his wife determined to limit their offspring to three. They have accordingly employed the above check for seven or eight years; have had no more children; and have been rewarded for **their** prudence by finding their situation and prospects improving every year. He confirmed an opinion I have already expressed, by stating, that custom completely reconciled him to any slight privation he might at first have felt. **I asked him, whether** his neighbours generally followed the same practice. He replied, that he **could** not tell; for he had not thought it prudent to speak with any but his own relations on the subject, **one or** two of whom, he knew, had profited by his advice, and afterwards expressed to him their gratitude **for the important information.**

It is unnecessary farther to multiply instances. **The** fact that this check is in common practice, and **universally** known to be efficacious, in France, **is alone sufficient** evidence **of its practicability and safety.**

I can readily imagine, that there are men, who, in part from temperament, but much more from the continued habit of unrestrained indulgence, may have so little command over their passions, as to find difficulty in practising it; and some, it may be, who will declare it to be impossible. If any there be to whom it *is* impossible, (which I very much doubt,) I am at least con**vinced** that the number **is** exceedingly small; not a fiftieth part of those who may at first *imagine* such to be their case.

I may add, that *partial* withdrawal, though recommended in a letter published in Carlile's Republican, is not an infallible preventive of conception.

Other modes of prevention have been employed,* but this is at once the most simple, and the most efficacious; the only one, or nearly so, employed by the cultivated among European nations; and the only one I here venture to recommend. From all I have heard, as well from physicians as from private individuals, it is, as regards health, at the least, perfectly innocent: it has been even said to produce upon the human system an effect similar to that of temperance in diet; **but** whether there be truth in this hypothesis I know not. As re-regards any moral impropriety in its use, enough, methinks, has already been said, to convince all except those who *will* not be convinced, that to employ it, in all cases where prudence or the well-being of our companions requires it, is an act of practical **virtue.**

It may be said, and said truly, that this check places **the power chiefly in the hands of** the man, and not,

---

* One of these modes, that of the sponge, is particularly recommended in Carlile's "Every Woman's Book." I do not allude to it in the text: because I believe it to be of doubtful efficacy; and, more certainly, physically disagreeable in its effects; and because I feel convinced, that the selfish of either sex will adopt *no* expedient, while the well-disposed **will** adopt the best in preference. Carlile supposes this to be the check common among **the** cultivated classes in France. In this he is mistaken. It is not employed, **and scarcely** known there. Had Carlile had **an opportunity of conversing with French physicians,** he would **have satisfactorily ascertained this fact.**

I also pass over all allusion to the *baudruche*, which is every way inconvenient, and is chiefly used to guard against syphilis. I do not write to facilitate, but, **on the contrary, effectually to** prevent, the degrading intercourse of which it is intended to obviate the penalty.

where it ought to be, in those of the woman. She, who is the sufferer, is not secured against the culpable carelessness, or perhaps the deliberate selfishness, of him who goes free and unblamed, whatever may happen. To this, the reply is, that the best and only effectual defence for women is to refuse connexion with any man *void of honour*. An (almost omnipotent) public opinion would thus be speedily formed; one of immense moral utility, by means of which the man's social reputation would be placed, as it should be, in the keeping of women, whose moral tact and nice discrimination in such matters is far superiour to ours. How mighty and how beneficent the power which such an influence might exert, and how essentially and rapidly it might conduce to the gradual, but thorough extirpation of those selfish vices, legal and illegal, which now disgrace and brutify our species, it is difficult even to imagine.

In the silent, but resistless progress of human improvement, such a change is fortunately inevitable. We are gradually emerging from the night of blind prejudice and of brutal force; and, day by day, rational liberty and cultivated refinement, win an accession of power. Violence yields to benevolence, compulsion to kindness, the letter of law to the spirit of justice: and, day by day, men and women become more willing, and better prepared, to entrust the most sacred duties (social as well as political) more to good feeling and less to idle form— more to **moral** and less to legal keeping.

It is no question whether such reform will come: no human power **can arrest** its **progress**. How slowly or how rapidly it may come, *is* a question; and depends, in some degree, on adventitious circumstances. Should this little **book** prove one among the number of circumstances to accelerate, however slightly, that progress, its author will be repaid, ten times over, for any trifling labour it may have cost him.

In conclusion, it may be useful to state to the reader the following facts:—A knowledge of this and other checks to population has been, for many years, extensively disseminated in most of the populous towns in Great Britain; not only through the medium of "Every Woman's Book," but, previously to its publication, by hundreds of thousands of handbills, which were gratuitously distributed from benevolent motives. The men who were first instrumental in making them known in England, are all elderly men, fathers of families of children grown up to be men and women: men of unimpeachable integrity, and of first rate moral character; many of them men of science, and some of them known as the first political economists and philanthropists of the age. Besides the allusion to the subject already given from the Encyclopedia Britannica, it is adverted to in Mill's " Elements of Political Economy ;" in Place's " Illustrations of the Principle of Population ;" in Thompson's " Distribution of Wealth," and probably in other works with which I am unacquainted. It was also (disguisedly) broached in several English newspapers, and was preached in lectures to the labouring classes, by a most benevolent man, at Leeds. I do not believe the subject has ever been touched upon, in one single instance, except by men of irreproachable moral character, and generally of high standing in society. The chief difference between this little treatise, and the allusions made by the distinguished authors above mentioned, is, that what public opinion would only permit them to insinuate, I venture to say plainly.

My readers may implicitly depend on the accuracy of

the facts I have stated. Though, in the present state of public opinion, **I may** not, **for** obvious reasons, give *names* in proof, **yet** it is evident that I **cannot** have the shadow of **a** motive to mislead or deceive. I shall consider it a favour if any individuals who can **adduce,** *from personal experience,* facts connected **with this subject, will** communicate them **to me.**

Note. **The** enlightened Condorcet, in his well-known **"** *Esquisse des progres de l'esprit humain,*" **very** distinctly **alludes to the** safety and facility **with** which population might be restrained, **"if reason should but keep** pace with the arts and sciences, and if **the** idle prejudices of superstition should cease to shed over human **morals an austerity** corrupting and degrading, not purifying or elevating." See his *Esquisse, pages* 285 to 288, *Paris* Ed. 1822.

Malthus (see his *"Essays on Population,"* Book 3, *chap.* 1) "professes not to understand" the French philosopher. No Frenchman could misunderstand him.

CHAPTER VII.

CONCLUDING REMARKS.

That most practical of philosophers, Franklin, interprets chastity to mean, *the regulated and strictly **temperate satisfaction, without injury to others, of those desires which** are natural **to all healthy** adult **beings**.* In this sense, chastity is the first of virtues, and one most rarely practised, either by young men or by married persons, even when the latter most scrupulously conform to the letter of the law.*

The promotion of such chastity is the chief object of the present work. It is all-important for the welfare of our race, that the reproductive instinct should never be selfishly indulged; never gratified at the expense of the well-being of our companions. A man who, in this matter, will not consult, with scrupulous deference, the slightest wishes of the other sex; a man who will ever put his desires in competition with theirs, and who will prize more highly the pleasure he receives than that he may be capable of bestowing—such a man appears to me, in the essentials of character, a brute. The brutes commonly seek the satisfaction of their propensities with straight-forward selfishness, and never calculate whether their companions are gratified or teased by their impor-

* My father, Robert Owen's definition of chastity is also an excellent one: "Prostitution, Sexual intercourse *without* affection; Chastity, Sexual intercourse *with* affection.

tunities. Man cannot assimilate his nature more closely to theirs, than by imitating them in this.

Again. **There is no instinct in** regard to which strict temperance is more essential. All our animal desires have hitherto occupied an undue share **of human** thoughts; **but** none more generally than this. **The** imaginations of the young and the passions of the adult are inflamed by mystery or excited by restraint, and a full half of all the thoughts and intrigues of **the world** has a direct reference to this single **instinct. Even those who, like the Shakers,** " crucify the flesh," are not the less occupied by it in their secret thoughts; as the Shaker writings themselves may afford proof. Neither human institutions nor human prejudices can destroy the instinct. Strange it is, that men should not be content rationally to control, and wisely to regulate it.

It is a question of passing importance, " How may it best be **regulated ?" Not by a Shaker vow of** monkish chastity. Assuredly not by the world's favourite regulator, ignorance. No. Do we wish to bring this instinct under easy government, and to assign it only its due rank among human sentiments? Then let us culti**vate** the intellect, let us exercise the body, let us usefully occupy the time, of every human being. What is it gives to passion its sway, and to **desires their empire,** now? It is vacancy of mind; it is listlessness of body; it is idleness. A cultivated race **are never sensual; a hardy race are** seldom **love-sick; an industrious race have no time to be sentimental. Develope** the moral sentiments, and they will govern the physical **instincts.** Occupy the mind and body usefully, intellectually; and the propensities will obtain **that care** and time only which **they merit.** Upon any **other** principle we may doctor **poor human** nature **for ever, and** shall **only prove our-**

selves empirics in the end. Mortifications, vestal vows, mysteries, bolts and bars, prudish prejudices—these are all quack-medicines; and are only calculated to prostrate the strength and spirits, or to heighten the fever, of the patient. If we will dislodge error and passion from the mind, we must replace them by something better. They say that a vacuum cannot exist in nature. Least of all can it exist in the human mind. Empty it of one folly, cure it of one vice, and another flows in to fill the vacancy, unless it find it already occupied by intellectual exercise and common sense.

Husbands and fathers! study Franklin's definition of chastity. Your fears, your jealousies, have hitherto been on the stretch to watch and guard: reflect whether it be not pleasanter and better, to enlighten and trust.

Honest ascetics! you have striven to mortify the flesh; ask yourselves whether it be not wiser to control it. You have sought to crucify the body; consider whether it be not more effectual to cultivate the mind. Have you succeeded in spiritualizing your secret thoughts? If not, enquire whether all human propensities, duly governed, be not a benefit and a blessing to the nature in which they are inherent.

Human beings, of whatever sex or class! examine dispassionately and narrowly the influence which the control here recommended will produce throughout society. Reflect whether it will not lighten the burdens of one sex, while it affords scope for the exercise of the best feelings of the other. Consider whether its tendency be not benignant and elevating; conducive to the exercise of practical virtue, and to the permanent welfare of the human race.

APPENDIX

TO THE FIFTH EDITION.

Reception of the Work by the Public. Opinion of a talented Author. Opinion of a Physician and Professor. Letter from a Mechanic. The work never intended as a political Panacea. Transmission of hereditary disease. Letter on the subject. Letter from a French gentleman. Physiological argument in favour of temperance. Experience of two members of the Society of Friends. Objection of J. W. Objections by a physician of Indiana. **Answer to them.**

New-York, June 25, 1831.

SEVEN months have not yet elapsed since the first publication of "Moral Physiology;" and already I am called upon to prepare a fifth edition. If I am pleased (as what author is not) to see that my labours are not unappreciated by the public, I am also reminded of the additional obligations I lie under, to render the little treatise as complete and as free from error and inaccuracy as possible.

I have therefore carefully revised the work, and made such amendments as have suggested themselves during these seven months. And as, in the course of that time, I have received a multitude of communications (some verbal, but chiefly by letter) on the subject in question, I shall here add, in the shape of Appendix, such extracts from, and comments on, a few of these, as seem to me interesting and useful.

I expected much opprobrium from the work; and have been not a little surprised to find my expectations most agreeably disappointed. Never, in my life, have I written any thing that so nearly united the suffrages of all whose opinion I care for, or which has been suffered to spread more quietly by our opponents. In this, these latter have acted wisely. Had they made any fuss about it, it would probably have been the Appendix to the *twentieth*, not to the *fifth*, edition I should now be writing.

The sentiments of approval which have reached me from various quarters, have, in the expressive language of the Old Book, "strengthened my hands and encouraged my heart;" for, though the world's opinion be worth little, there are individuals in it whose opinion is worth much; and though a consciousness of rectitude may support a man against *all* opinions, yet it is pleasant to find, now and then, in one's progress, concurrent sentiments from those we esteem.

I imagine that it may afford similar encouragement, in a degree, to any of my readers who may chance to approve what they read, if I quote for them a few of these opinions. And, first, I select for the purpose two, which come from men both known to me, as to the American public, only by their writings. Could I give the names of the writers, these would be sufficient to secure for their opinions a weight which no anonymous sentiments can obtain. But, in the present state of public opinion, I do not feel myself, for obvious reasons, at liberty to do so. My readers must therefore be content to take my word for it, that both the writers are gentlemen who have displayed in their works talents of a high order, and whose personal acquaintance I should consider it an honour to make.

I extract from the first letter the following:

"I am greatly obliged to you for sending me your 'Moral Physiology.' I have read it with pleasure and instruction. I see not why you should anticipate censure, from any quarter, for its publication. It contains no sentiment or doctrine which strikes me unfavourably, or which any person could wish suppressed. Had the same thoughts occurred to me, I should have entertained them, and possibly published them, without the least suspicion of offence to delicacy or good morals.

"I fully concur with you, that truth can do the world no harm. Nor do I doubt that he should be deemed a benefactor, (even an exceedingly great benefactor,) who can teach man how to limit his powers of reproduction without abridging his enjoyments."

Again, the same correspondent says:

"The value of the power to limit offspring, is, I think, very separable from any theory which involves consequences arising from the extent of population which the earth can sustain. The limitation is a matter which concerns the present comfort of individuals, in their private capacity; while the extent of the earth's ultimate fecundity concerns only the thoughts or speculatists and politicians. I say this, because I am not troubled by the spectre of Malthus."

This appears to me an enlightened, and also a very practical view of the subject. The political economy of the question ought ever to be kept separate from its moral bearings. The consequences involved by the former, are distant, and may be called theoretical; while those resulting from the latter, are immediate, and of daily recurrence in practice. If there were no tendency whatever in the human race to increase beyond its present numbers, the question would still be one of vital interest, and the consequences it **involves would** still be **of surpassing** importance to man in his social and domestic relations. **The more I reflect on** the subject, the more thoroughly convinced **I am,** *that man can never attain to any thing like social cultivation, without a knowledge of the means to limit, at pleasure and without much sacrifice of enjoyment, his power of reproduction.* And I cannot but think that all who have **seen much of the** civilized world, and carefully traced out the various causes of the vices and miseries that pervade it, will, upon reflection, **concur with me in the opinion.**

The second writer of whom I spoke (an eminent physician and professor) says:

" I have received your **' Moral** Physiology.' Your **boldness** and **independence** are entitled **to** great respect. It is a very important question, and ought to be brought forward, that the public opinion concerning it may be based on the only proper ground, full and free and patient public discussion. Your method of handling **the** subject **I** approve. *Piace*, the **political** economist, suggests the remedy **more boldly than any other."**

The next **communication from which I shall copy is** from **a young man of excellent character, living in a** neighbouring **state, and now one of the conductors of a popular** periodical. After suggesting **to** me the propriety **of re-publishing** some English works now out of print, he proceeds as **follows:**

"―――, *February* 23, 1831.

" Had I not been addressing you upon another subject, I should not have ventured to obtrude on you my small meed of approbation, due to your last work; but I cannot let slip this opportunity of endeavouring to express how much I feel indebted to you for its publication.

"To know how I am so indebted, it is necessary you should also know something of my situation in life: and when it is described, it is perhaps a description of the situation of two thirds of the journeymen mechanics of this country.

"I have been married nearly three years, and am the father of two children. Having nothing to depend upon but my own industry, you will readily acknowledge that I had reason to look forward with at least some degree of disquietude to the prospect of an increasing family and reduced wages; apparently the inevitable lot of the generality of working men. Under these circumstances, I saw W. Jackson's article in the Delaware Free Press; but my feelings as a freeman (nominally) revolted at it, and I must say that I felt greatly pleased when I found that his system did not meet your approbation. You had spoken upon the subject, but, like the Nazarene Reformer, you spoke in parables. 'Every Woman's Book' I could not see; and, had not Dr. Gibbons afforded me an example of how much you might be misrepresented, I might have been tempted to believe the slanders circulated regarding you.

"I had apparently nothing left but to let matters take their own course, when your 'Moral Physiology' made its appearance.

"I read it; and a new scene of existence seemed to open before me. I found myself, in this all important matter, a free agent, and, in a degree, the arbiter of my own destiny. I could have said to you, as Selim said to Hassan,

'Thou'st hewed a mountain's weight from off my heart.'

My visions of poverty and future distress vanished; the present seemed gilded with new charms, and the future appeared no longer to be dreaded. But you can better imagine, than I describe, the revolution of my feelings.

"I have since endeavoured to circulate the little book as widely as my limited opportunities permit, and shall continue to do so, believing it to be the most useful work that has made its appearance since the publication of Paine's 'Common Sense;' and convinced that, by so doing, I shall render you the most acceptable return in my power to make for the benefit you have conferred upon me as an individual. G."

And here I may remark, that, though I expected my little book, in such individual cases as the above, to be (as it seems it has been) the means of diminishing the suffering which inequality of condition and the pressure of poverty bring upon men and women, yet I desire it to be distinctly understood, that I have never put it forward, and do not now put it forward, as a *remedy*, but only as a *palliative*, of political evils.* Were *all* poor parents (an unlikely case, however) thus to limit their offspring, it might, perchance, but furnish excuse and opportunity, in the present state of commercial competition, for their employers to lower their wages: for wages, as things are now arranged, too often sink nearly to the point of subsistence.† Economy in living is, like the parental foresight of which I have spoken, in itself an excellent thing; but he who expects, by the one recommendation or the other, to *cure* the ills of poverty, expects an effect from utterly inadequate causes. The root of the evil lies far deeper than this; and its remedy must be of a more radical nature. This is not the place, however, to enter on such a discussion. The great importance of the work I conceive to lie more in its *moral and social*, rather than in its *political*, bearings. It is addressed to each individual, rather as the member of a family, than the citizen of a state.

The next extract, from an inhabitant of Pennsylvania, I have selected chiefly as it furnishes a beautiful, and, alas! a rare, example, of that parental conscientiousness which scruples to impart existence where it cannot also impart the conditions necessary to render that existence happy. In this view, the control in question is indeed all-important. Were such virtue as this cultivated in mankind generally, how soon might the very seeds of disease die out among us, instead of bearing, as now, their poison-fruit from generation to generation! and how far might human beings, in succeeding ages, surpass their forefathers in strength, in health, and in beauty!

---

* See page 31 of the work itself.

† This, however, applies, at the present time, rather to Great Britain than to this country.

This view of the subject is to the physiologist, to the philosopher, to every friend of human improvement, a most interesting one. "So long," to use the words of an eloquent lecturer, now in this city, "as the tainted stream is unhesitatingly transmitted through the channel of nature, from parent to offspring, so long will the text be verified which 'visits the sins of the fathers on the children, even to the third and fourth generation.'" And so long, I would add, will mankind (wise and successful whenever there is question of improving the animal races) be blind in perceiving, and listless in securing, that far nobler object, the physical, and thereby (in a measure) the mental and moral improvement of our own.

I may seem an enthusiast—but so let me seem then—when I express my conviction, that there is not greater physical disparity between the dullest, shaggiest race of dwarf draught horses, and the fiery-spirited and silken-haired Arabian, than between man degenerate as he is, and man perfected as he might be: and though mental cultivation in this counts for much, yet organic melioration is an influential—is an *indispensable* necessary.

Here is the extract which led to these remarks:

"——, *March* 23, 1831.
* * * "I use no meat, unless eggs may be considered such; I drink neither tea, coffee, nor any thing more exciting than milk and water; and, like yourself, I am fully satisfied, having no craving after the luxuries of the table. With regard to 'Moral Physiology,' let the following facts speak:

"I was born of poor parents, and early left an orphan. When of age, though my circumstances promised poorly for the support of a family, I desired to marry, knowing that a good wife would greatly add to my happiness. The check spoken of in your book (withdrawal) presented itself to my mind. And for seven years that I have now been married, I have continued to practise it. I was successful in business, and acquired the means of maintaining a family; but still I have refrained, because my constitution is such an one as I think a parent ought not to transmit to his offspring. I prefer refraining from giving birth to sentient beings, unless I can give them those advantages, physical as well as moral and intellectual, which are essential to human happiness.

"One thing I have observed, that since I have adopted a simple diet, and laid by all artificial stimuli, not only is my health better, and my mind more clear, but I can abstain, at will, without injury or inconvenience, from sexual connexion for any length of time;* and this without having, in the least, lost any power in that respect. **T.**"

From the letter of an aged French gentleman, who holds a public office in the western country, I translate the following; and I would to heaven that every young man and woman in these United States could read it:

"I have read your little work with much interest, and desire that it may have a wide circulation, and that its recommendations may be adopted in practice. If you publish a third edition, I could wish that you would add a piece of advice of the greatest importance, especially to young married persons. Many women are ignorant, that, in the gratification of the reproductive instinct, the exhaustion to the man is much greater than to the woman: a fact most important to be known, the ignorance of which has caused more than one husband to forfeit his health, nay, his *life*. Tissot tells us, that the loss by an ounce of semen is equal to that by forty ounces of blood;† and that, in the case of the healthiest man, nature does not demand connexion oftener than once a month.‡

---

* We applaud, as a marvel, the continence of Scipio. Such continence—and amid circumstances far more trying—is habitually found (under no other restraint than that of public opinion) among the native Indians of our continent. A friend of mine, whose family was captured by a party of Mohawk Indians some fifty years ago, informed me, that four young women (two of them of considerable beauty) who were captured on that occasion, were not once, during a residence of several years, addressed, even with the remotest degree of sexual importunity, by an Indian, old or young, though living with them in the same wigwam. These young women were the near relatives of the friend who related this fact to me; and it was from their own lips he obtained it. Yet these were savages!

Such scrupulous regard to the feelings of others, would be a matter of too universal prevalence among us even to cause remark, or call forth commendation, were it not for the artificial stimuli, and as artificial restraints, which fashion and law make common among us. R. D. O.

† This, of course, must be rather a matter of conjecture and approximation, than of accurate calculation. R. D. O.

‡ And I doubt whether she *permits* it, without more or less of injury, to the average of constitutions, oftener than once a week. Certain I am, that any young

"How many young spouses, loving their husbands tenderly and disinterestedly, if they were but informed of these facts, would watch over and preserve their partners' healths, instead of exciting them to over-indulgence.

"I send you a copy of Italian verses, appropriate, like the German stanza you have quoted in your work, to the above remarks:

> 'Merta gli allori al crine
> Chi scende in campo armato,
> Chi a cento squadre a lato,
>   Impallidir non sa:
> Ma più gloria ha nel fronte
> Chi, alla ragion soggetto,
> D'un sconsigliato astello
>   Trionfator si fà.'* L. G."

I extract the following from my journal:

January 4, 1831.

A member of the Society of Friends, from the country, called at our office; he informed me that he had been married twenty years, had six children, and would probably have had twice as many, had he not practised withdrawal, which he found, in every instance, efficacious. By this means he made an interval of two or three years between the births of each of his children. Having at last a family of six, his wife earnestly desired to have no more; and on one occasion, when she imagined that the necessary precautions had been neglected, she shed tears at the prospect of again becoming pregnant. He

---

man who will carefully note and compare his sensations, will become convinced, that temperance positively forbids such indulgence, at any rate, more than twice a week; and that he trifles with his constitution who neglects the prohibition. How immeasurably important that parents should communicate to their sons, but especially to their daughters, facts like these! R. D. O.

* For the English reader, I have attempted the following imitation of the above lines:

> Crown his brows with laurel wreath,
> Who can tread the field of death—
> Tread—with armed thousands near—
> And know not what it is to fear.
> But greater far his meed of praise,
> Juster his claim to glory's bays,
> Who, true to reason's voice, to virtue's call,
> Conquers himself, the noblest deed of all! R. D. O.

said he knew, in his own neighbourhood, several married women who were rendered miserable on account of their continued pregnancy, and would have given any thing in the world to escape, but knew not how.

This gentleman corroborated the opinion I had suggested, (*page* 66,) that the habit of withdrawal had an influence similar to that of temperance in diet. He had found it, he said, much less exhausting than unrestrained indulgence.

Another gentleman, also belonging to the Society of Friends, has since confirmed to me (as a fact *positively proved* to him by personal experience) the above opinion. He likewise expressed his conviction, that the habit was greatly conducive to the preservation of those first, fresh feelings, (so beautiful, and, alas! so evanescent,) under which the married usually come together.

In reply to a correspondent, J. W., who cites a case of Priapism mentioned in a Medical Journal some eight or ten years since, and which pathological derangement he thinks was attributable to the habit of withdrawal, I would reply, that the concurrent testimony of all who can speak from experience on the subject, disproves, not of course the fact he cites, but the propriety of *attributing the effect produced to the cause in question*. Priapism, it is well known, is frequently caused by sexual excess; and was probably so caused in the case alluded to. Such excess is much less likely to take place, when withdrawal is practised, than during unrestrained indulgence.

It now remains for me to notice an important communication which I recently received from a medical gentleman residing in Indiana, for whose talents and character I entertain much respect. It regards the physiological portion of the work, which the writer, Dr. S——, thinks is altogether inaccurate.

He refers me to Burns', Denman's, and Dewee's Midwifery, and especially to an essay by Dr. Caldwell, of Transylvania University, on Generation, in proof, that all are *not* agreed that the semen must enter the uterus in order to effect impregnation. He instances a case published in the New-York Medical Repository, and another in the Western Quarterly Reporter, in which impregnation was effected, though immediately previous to the child's birth the vagina was found only large enough to admit a common knitting needle, and the medical attendant had, in consequence, to make an artificial passage. And he argues, on the authority of this and other instances where there existed such mechanical obstruction in the vagina, os tincæ or collum uteri, as to render the passage of the seminal fluid next to impossible, that that fluid does not enter the uterus at all, and, consequently, that the doctrine on which the whole work is founded, is physiologically false; and, as being false, is calculated to do much and cruel mischief. There are two chief theories, he says, now generally received on the subject, the *absorbent* and the *sympathetic;* according to both of which, all that appears absolutely necessary to impregnation is, that the semen should be deposited somewhere in the vagina; *perhaps*, to be taken up by a set of absorbent vessels, and by them conveyed to the ovum, which ovum is, in its turn, taken up by the fimbriated ends of the Fallopian tube, and thereby deposited in the uterus; *perhaps,* (but I confess this seems to me a very poetical theory,) merely to produce simultaneous and sympathetic action, thereby effecting the great and secret work of nature.

Now, my expression was, that "*almost* all physiologists are agreed, that the entrance of the sperm itself, *or of some volatile particles proceeding from it*, into the uterus, must precede conception."* The favourers of the *absorbent* theory will not, I presume, deny this; the few advocates of the *sympathetic*, may. Nor am I tenacious as regards any theory whatever, on a subject of which the arcana still remain shrouded in comparative mystery. Enough for my purpose, that the condition indispensable to reproduction is, (as Dr. S—— himself reminds us,) the deposition of the sperm in the vagina. The preventive suggested in "Moral Physiology," *positively* **precludes** the fulfil-

---

* In proof that I have not spoken unadvisedly on this subject, I may quote what, I believe, is now considered the highest authority:

"If the most recent works on Physiology are to be credited, the uterus, during impregnation, opens a little, draws in the semen by inspiration, and directs it to the ovarium by means of the Fallopian tubes, whose fimbriated extremity closely embraces that organ."—*Magendie*, p. 416, *Philad. Ed.*

See also *Blundell's* and *Haighton's* experiments on the rabbit, at Guy's hospital. See also *Spallanzani's* experiments.

ment of this condition; **and it could** only have been, I imagine, **by** confounding it with the partial expedient of which I have spoken, (*page* 66,) **that my** medical friend arrived at the conclusions **to which I have here alluded.**

The **only** argument which I conceive can be fairly urged against it by the physiologist, is that to which I **have adverted and** replied: (*last paragraph of page* 65.)

Having thus answered all the objections which have **hitherto** reached me, I conceive **it unnecessary to** lengthen **this** Appendix by farther quotations approbatory of the work, or corroborative of the facts it details. **Let** "Moral Physiology" abide the ordeal of **public examination;** if found wanting, **to be cast aside and forgotten;** but if deemed true and useful, **to be remembered and approved.**

NOTES BY THE PUBLISHER,

ON

ROBERT DALE OWEN'S MORAL PHYSIOLOGY.

Since this **work** was published by Robert **Dale** Owen, a flood of information **on** the subject has been shed upon the world; and France, **Germany,** Spain, and England, have **each been** made to contribute to the United States its share.

The following facts are now *positively* known: All female animals have their *courses;* and at such periods in the human species, an ovum or egg is brought down from the ovaries into the womb, through the Fallopian tubes (see plate). This ovum or egg arrives in the womb a day or two after the courses have ceased, but it may be longer. This is known from anatomy, and can be felt by an observing female, from a sense of weight and slight pain in the region of the Fallopian tubes, and across the lower abdomen. (See Dr. Hollick's Marriage Guide, article "Impregnation.") The egg in the womb is covered with a film, called the decedua, which retains it in the crown of the womb for some days: during that time the woman is liable to become pregnant, if she then indulge in sexuality, and to which act at that period Nature prompts the male by previous abstinence, and the female in common with all female animals. The ovum or egg remains in the womb or Fallopian tubes in all about fifteen days at most, but generally a less time; and, if unimpregnated, **corrupts and passes off** with a thin fluid, wetting the **adjacent external parts** with something like the white of an egg. This is followed by the escape of a *grayish-white clot,* as large as a pea or bean, which is found to be the ovum or egg, enveloped by the decedua; and this also may be *felt, seen,* and *examined,* by the attentive subject.

The mode of impregnation is **also** known. The semen of the male contains animalcules in bunches; these bunches develop rapidly, and ripen into individuals, in the **shape of an** *eel* (see engraving), with a propensity to dart or push forward. One of these, entering the ovum or egg, *that* becomes impregnated, if uncorrupted at that time. And such is the origin of a child, or man; and such was Napoleon, Charles XII., and Sir Isaac Newton.

Consequently, to avoid impregnation, we must prevent the entrance of the animalcule into the womb when the ovum or egg is present, or destroy it when there.

This object can be effected in various ways, any one or all of which it may be desirable to use in different circumstances. Avoid sexual union while liable to impregnation; that is, till after the escape of the ovum or egg. Withdrawal on the part of the male, before emission, is an effectual prevention; but it is only practicable with safety by the male in the *decline* of life, when the semen is deposited slowly: in youth and mature manhood it is ejected promptly and with force; it is therefore difficult to control.

A partial withdrawal or deposite of semen within the vagina (see plate), but not near the womb (which is situated at the extremity of the vagina, or passage to the womb), is safe, if the semen be removed by a syringe immediately afterwards.

The use of the syringe with cold water is effective immediately after coition; but rheumatism of the womb *may be* a consequence of this preventive. Nor will any ingredient, such as soda, prevent the consequence.

A *complete preventive* is the use of the syringe with water and a little alcohol or common whiskey, &c., as strong as convenient, which experience will discover. A folded cloth or sheet may be laid under the subject, and the remedy applied while in bed, with no inconvenience; and this may be relied upon, for the alcohol destroys the animalcules. Should the alcohol be unpleasant from its strength, the application of cold water will correct the error, and in *such circumstances* be perfectly safe.

Most books on this subject reserve a secret, for which you have to remit a dollar. This is quackery. The foregoing may be relied upon; it is all that is requisite, and has been thoroughly tested.

The drugs employed by the medical faculty are opium, prussic acid, iodine (and strychnine by the French). We do not recommend them. Other remedies have been mentioned in the body of the work.

We subjoin a list of **modern works in the English language** upon this and collateral subjects, which may be consulted with advantage, **and which can** be **had at our** office:—

> Moral Physiology, a Plain Treatise on the Population Question, with Notes by the Publisher, G. VALE; embracing all that is now known upon the subject, and illustrated by Anatomical Engravings. Paper, 37½ cts.; boards .... $ .50
> Hollick's Male Organs............................ 1.00
> Hollick's Matron's Manual........................ 1.00
> Hollick's Marriage Guide 1.00
> **Nichols's Esoteric Anthropology**................. 1.00
> Nichols on Marriage.............................. 1.00

Office, 5 CHATHAM SQUARE, NEW YORK.

NOTES ON THE TEXT.

ONANISM.—The **vice of onanism, or self-pollution, is** practised by **both sexes. The chief injury is in the nervous** irritability often **kept up for a long while, and frequently** repeated by those who **know not the consequences.** The loss of semen **in the male is much easier repaired than the** shattered nerves, **occasioned** by protracted excitement.—See page 42.

THE BAUDRUCHE.—The *baudruche* or *condum* is a cover or case to the male organ, made of fine skin **or silk,** and is used, as the author remarks, both **to prevent conception** and disease by contagion. As we cannot prevent vice, we see **no reason** for not abating **the consequent misery.** The free use of water, especially if a little soda be mixed, immediately after coition, will generally prevent the effects of contagion; but its frequent use with the alkali named might be injurious.

We have seen a new article, called "The French Safe," made of India rubber and gutta percha, which appears admirably adapted to the object proposed. It is more durable, and less expensive. This has been introduced to us by Dr. Ralph Darby.—p. 66.

CONCEPTION.—A wife can discover by a little attention when an emission is about to take place, and can therefore guard against the consequences, if necessary; or the use of a sponge before, or of a female syringe afterwards, or both, will give her complete control.

There is a fact connected with this subject, though known to many in practice, which has yet escaped the vigilance of previous writers; while anatomy has served to mislead, because it can be practised only on the dead. On dissection of the female organs, the mouth of the womb is seen to be nearly closed, scarcely admitting a small wire, and hence some have supposed that the male organ could not enter, and these have doubted even if the semen, when ejected, could force an entrance into the womb; they therefore supposed that absorption took place in some mysterious manner. The fact is, that the neck of the womb comes down in the act of coition, and the mouth opens, at least sufficiently to receive the end of a finger: and this coming down of the neck of the womb is connected with the extreme sensibility sometimes felt; and at those times the proof can be most easily obtained.—p. 67.

SEXUAL CAPACITY.—This is so various in different individuals, both male and female, that no rule can have a general application. What would be excess in one, is harmless in another. A modification in the marriage laws, where much discrepancy exists, is the natural remedy.—p 80.

☞ This work is therefore recommended to those who require its aid, as complete and without reserve. Nothing is kept back; all of any use, that is known, is given, and the information is all-sufficient; while the price will place it in the hands of the poor as well as of the rich, a desirable object for every useful work.

G. V.

NEW YORK, *October*, 1858.

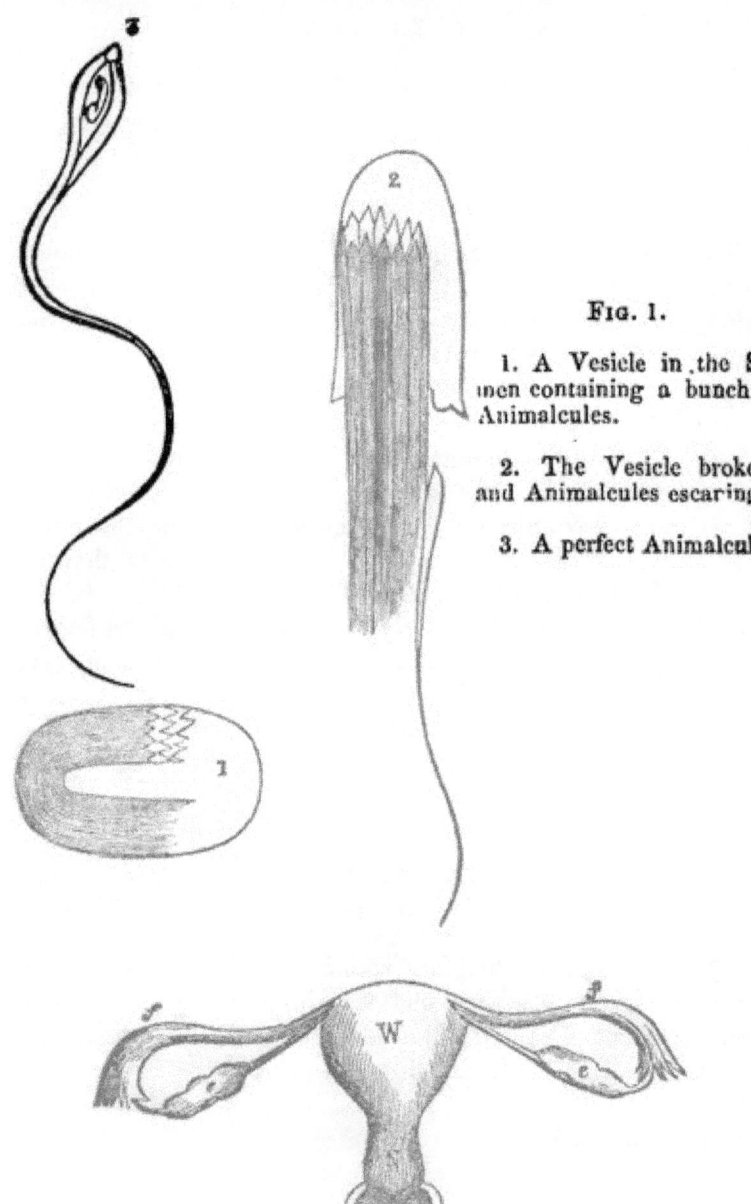

FIG. 1.

1. A Vesicle in the Semen containing a bunch of Animalcules.

2. The Vesicle broken, and Animalcules escaping.

3. A perfect Animalcule.

FIG. 2.—*f, f*, Fallopian Tubes.—*e, e*, Ovaries or Eggs.—*W*, Womb.—*N*, Neck of the Womb.—*C*, Passage into the Womb or Vagina.

www.ingramcontent.com/pod-product-compliance
Lightning Source LLC
Chambersburg PA
CBHW020259090426
42735CB00009B/1147